**LEGENDS
LEADERS
PIONEERS**

INTERVIEWS FROM THE SOCIETY FOR VASCULAR SURGERY'S HISTORY PROJECT WORK GROUP

Chairmen: James S.T. Yao 2010–2018   Walter J. McCarthy 2018–2023

LEGENDS
LEADERS
PIONEERS

SURGEONS WHO BUILT VASCULAR SURGERY

Foreword by Norman Rich

LEGENDS LEADERS PIONEERS: *Surgeons Who Built Vascular Surgery*
© Copyright 2024, The Society for Vascular Surgery
38678 Eagle Way Chicago IL 60678   svshistoryproject@gmail.com

All rights reserved. No part of this book may be used or reproduced in any manner whatsoever without written permission from the publisher, except in the case of brief quotations in critical articles and reviews.
Paperback First Edition   ISBN 13: 978-1-956872-50-7
Hardcover First Edition   ISBN 13: 978-1-956872-74-3

AMIKA PRESS   466 Central AVE #23 Northfield IL 60093   847 920 8084
info@amikapress.com   Available for purchase on amikapress.com
Edited by John K. Manos.
Designed and typeset by Sarah Koz. Set in Slimbach, designed by Robert Slimbach, 1987. Titles in Benton Sans Condensed Medium, designed by Cyrus Highsmith and Tobias Frere-Jones, 2000. Thanks to Nathan Matteson.

For James S.T. Yao

Contents

xi Foreword
xiii Acknowledgments
xvi Introduction

2 Enrico Ascher, MD

4 Ronald J. Baird, MD

6 William H. Baker, MD

8 Panagiotis E. Balas, MD

10 Wylie F. Barker, MD

12 Jonathan D. Beard, MD

14 Jean-Pierre Becquemin, MD

16 Ramon Berguer, MD, PhD

18 F. William Blaisdell, MD

20 Jan D. Blankensteijn, MD, PhD

22 Jan S. Brunkwall, MD

24 Jacob Buth, MD

26 Allan D. Callow, MD

28 Richard P. Cambria, MD

30 Piergiorgio Cao, MD

32 Stephen W.K. Cheng, MD

34 Timothy A.M. Chuter, MD

36 G. Patrick Clagett, MD

38 Alexander Whitehill Clowes, MD

40 John E. Connolly, MD

42 Denton A. Cooley, MD

44 Jack L. Cronenwett, MD

46 Herbert Dardik, MD

48 Richard H. Dean, MD

50 Michael DeBakey, MD

54 James Arville DeWeese, MD

57 Edward B. Diethrich, MD

59 Jeanne Doyle, RN
    Victoria Fahey, RN

60 Ben Eiseman, MD

63 José Fernandes e Fernandes, MD

65 Thomas J. Fogarty, MD

67 Julie Ann Freischlag, MD

69 Peter Gloviczki, MD

72 Olivier Goëau-Brissonnière, MD, PhD

74 Jerry Goldstone, MD

76 Richard M. Green, MD

78 Lazar J. Greenfield, MD

80 Roger M. Greenhalgh, MD

82 John P. Harris, MD

84 Norman R. Hertzer, MD

86 Larry H. Hollier, MD

88 Jimmy F. Howell, MD

90 Anthony M. Imparato, MD

92 Julius H. Jacobson II, MD

95 K. Wayne Johnston, MD

97 K. Craig Kent, MD

99 Robert L. Kistner, MD

101 Peter F. Lawrence, MD

104 Christos D. Liapis, MD

106 Frank W. LoGerfo, MD

108 William T. Maloney

110 John A. Mannick, MD

113 Kenneth L. Mattox, MD

116 James May, MD

118 D. Craig Miller, MD

120 Frans L. Moll, MD

122 Wesley S. Moore, MD

125 Hassan Najafi, MD

128 George P. Noon, MD

130 John L. Ochsner, MD

133 Thomas F. O'Donnell, Jr., MD

135 Juan Carlos Parodi, MD

138 William H. Pearce, MD

141 Bruce A. Perler, MD

143 Anatoly V. Pokrovsky, MD

146 Jean-Baptiste Ricco, MD

149 Norman M. Rich, MD

152 Thomas S. Riles, MD

154 Charles Granville Rob, MD

157 Harris B. Shumacker Jr., MD

160 Gregorio A. Sicard, MD

163 Anton N. Sidawy, MD

165 Robert B. Smith III, MD

167 Frank C. Spencer, MD

170 James C. Stanley, MD

172 Ronald J. Stoney, MD

175 Jonathan B. Towne, MD

177 Frank J. Veith, MD

180 J. Leonel Villavicencio, MD

182 Shenming Wang, MD, PhD

184 Milton Weinberg, MD

187 Jock R. Wheeler, MD

190 Anthony Dunster Whittemore, MD

193 John H.N. Wolfe, MD

195 James S.T. Yao, MD, PhD

198 Christopher K. Zarins, MD

201 Robert M. Zwolak, MD

203 Appendix I
    204 Kenneth J. Cherry Jr., MD
    206 Calvin B. Ernst, MD
    208 Mark K. Eskandari, MD
    210 Roger T. Gregory, MD
    212 Melina R. Kibbe, MD
    214 Richard A. Lynn, MD
    216 Walter J. McCarthy III, MD
    218 Jan Muller

220 Appendix II

Foreword

Surgeons have respect and love for history. This is particularly true for vascular surgeons as this book will identify and emphasize. The history of vascular surgery is that of a relatively new surgical specialty. This was detailed by James Yao, Roger Gregory and Norman Rich in their article, "Interviews with Pioneers of Vascular Surgery" published under the auspices of the Society for Vascular Surgery (SVS) in 2012 in the *Journal of Vascular Surgery*.

Several notable histories of vascular surgery in the 20th century are available. Harris Shumacker wrote about the early years of the SVS in his book, *The Society for Vascular Surgery, A History: 1945–1983*. At the 50th anniversary of the SVS, Calvin Ernest and Yao covered the history from 1946 to 1996, at which time Michael DeBakey and Shumacker were interviewed on video. In the Joint Council of the SVS and the North American Chapter of the International Cardiovascular Society, from 1976 to 1986 Rich had the responsibility for reporting on the development of the increasing number of regional vascular societies, with each society proudly outlining its history. Additional historical references come from the book by Andrew Dale, completed by James DeWeese and George Johnson, entitled *Band of Brothers: Creators of Modern Vascular Surgery*, which is made up of edited transcripts from tape-recorded interviews with 37 pioneer vascular surgeons. Much information also comes from a section in the *Journal of Vascular Surgery*, edited by Rich, entitled *Vignettes in Vascular Surgery*. This was at the time when the co-chief editors were Anton Sidawy and Bruce Perler. Additionally, there is valuable information in a book published in 1989 by Stephen G. Friedman entitled *A History of Vascular Surgery*.

Yao called Rich several times in late 2011 proposing that they invite Roger Gregory to join them with Ernst as a consultant to establish the SVS History

Project Work Group (Work Group) to review and record the experiences of pioneers in vascular surgery. This was supported by Richard Cambria and Peter Gloviczki, representing the SVS leadership at that time. The first interviews were in 2011, including five in Chicago in December 2021, during the annual Northwestern Vascular Symposium. Yao recruited Jan Muller as videographer—who helped ensure the highest professional quality of the interviews—that were placed online under the SVS website, with the plan to write a book on the history of vascular surgery. Soon thereafter, it was decided that additional colleagues should be added to expand the effort, and these initially included Kenneth Cherry, William Baker, Mark Eskandari, Melina Kibbe, Peter Lawrence, Walter McCarthy and William Pearce. Toward the later years of the project, John (Jeb) Hallett, Richard Lynn and James Menzoian were also recruited. McCarthy assumed the Work Group chairmanship from Yao in 2018, with the enthusiastic support of Yao, carrying on the outstanding effort.

These interviews of world leaders in vascular surgery and this book ensure that the history of the exciting development of vascular surgery is available to future generations. It is dedicated to the memory of Yao, as a testament to the innovative and tenacious leadership effort of Dr./Professor James S.T. Yao of Chicago and Northwestern University.

Norman M. Rich, MD
COL, MC, USA (Ret)
Bethesda, Maryland
January 24, 2023

Acknowledgments

The History Project Work Group video interviews, and subsequently this book, are a logical progression from the 50th anniversary historical review completed by the Society for Vascular Surgery (SVS). The 50th anniversary presentation had been prepared for the 1997 annual SVS meeting and had been chaired by James Yao and Calvin Ernst. After a number of years had passed, a new historical review, centering around video interviews was envisioned. With James Yao as the leader, Norman Rich, Calvin Ernst and Roger Gregory share responsibility for initiating this current effort in 2011. When the project was initially proposed, Peter Gloviczki and Richard Cambria were vascular society leaders, and we thank them for their encouragement and indeed for their permission to go ahead, including assuring funding for the work from the SVS. Funding, first for the video interview production and editing, then more recently for this book, has continued over the last twelve years through the SVS. All of the funding was used for the videographer's time and travel expenses. None of the interviewers received any reimbursement. Related to this book, the SVS holds not only the copyright but also the right to any subsequent royalties.

The SVS executive directors and staffs played a critical role in achieving a successful conclusion of this very long-term project. In 2011, Rebecca Maron was the executive director and provided this leadership and subsequently, Kenneth Slaw has continued with guidance and support.

Nearly all of the video interviews and technical editing were accomplished by Jan Muller. Mr. Muller also did much background research and biographical writing. Without his enthusiastic, persistent effort and many talents, the project would never have been completed.

Each of the surgeons who conducted interviews contributed much of their valuable time to researching and then meeting with the vascular surgeons to be interviewed. Their enthusiasm and confidence in the overall importance of the undertaking greatly propelled the project. The tremendous advantage of having individuals very familiar with the topic conduct the interviews is one of the strong suits of this project. The interviewers, particularly the more senior ones, provided much of the gravitas that allowed the project to live on despite its long horizon. We also wish to thank those who were interviewed. Every one of them provided remarkably detailed, personal and thought-provoking interviews.

Nearly every video is accompanied by music composed by John Yao, James and Louise Yao's son, who is a trombone player and a professional musician.

The leader among the interviewers was Roger Gregory, who conducted more of the interviews than anyone else and even years before this current project, had interviewed prominent surgeons on his own. His contribution cannot be overstated, and the fundamental style of the interviews is a reflection of his own guidelines, which he taught each of the interviewers. His instructions influenced the structure and flow of nearly every interview:

1. The interview should be conducted not to hear the interviewers talk about themselves;
2. each interview should be designed to stand as a coherent entity and thus needs a brief introduction and explanation of the overall project;
3. interviews usually should begin with, "tell us about where you grew up and about your family life;"
4. then, "tell us about your education and surgical training;"
5. next inquire, "who were your mentors early on and throughout life;"
6. and finally, explore multiple other areas, such as:
   - what operations did you perform,
   - which were your favorites,
   - what were your most important accomplishments,
   - what do you think about the future of training vascular surgeons,
   - what do you think about the structure of the vascular societies,
   - what are your thoughts regarding healthcare in the United States,
   - tell us a bit about your family life and your activities besides medicine,
   - and do you have advice for younger people contemplating a career in vascular surgery?

The funding for this actual book was approved by SVS Executive Director Kenneth Slaw in November, 2022 and the authors desire to record our thanks to him for this. My biographical writing, expansion of existing material and fact-checking was begun in earnest once funding was approved. Most of the video interviews were already accompanied by biographical material, some extensive and some very brief. Each of these biographies had been written previously either by this author or by James Yao along with Jan Muller. The facts and verbiage for the final biographies have drawn greatly from curriculum vitae, personal biographies sent by the interviewees, key published papers, obituaries, quotes from the actual interviews, online research, and in some cases, biographies and autobiographies. Every effort was made to make all of the sentence structures original. The authors apologize for whatever small amount may have been transferred verbatim by the multiple authors over several years.

Critical to the success of this book was the selection of the editor and the publishing house. We selected the talented editor, John Manos, who had previously produced an historical textbook about surgery at Cook County Hospital for James Yao. His company, Amika Press, is well suited for this project, and Mr. Manos' suggestion of publication on demand through Amazon was a critical decision. Mr. Manos' editorial skills and overall support are greatly appreciated. Over the last twelve months, the author's wife, Mary McCarthy, reviewed each biography for sentence structure and grammar immediately after it was written, greatly enhancing the readability.

Sad circumstances bring me to write these acknowledgments by myself in the absence of James Yao following his death on December 20, 2022. He was the one with the original vision for this project, and used his well-known enthusiastic leadership, organizational skills and optimism to assure that the work would be completed.

Walter McCarthy, MD
Chicago, Illinois
October 25, 2023

Updated information can be sent
to svshistoryproject@gmail.com

Introduction

The motivation for proceeding with the vascular surgery history project and eventually, this book, was that there was a remarkable story to tell. The technology and surgical awareness to not just ligate but to repair and reconstruct human blood vessels is truly something new in the long history of surgery. Despite a few earlier, isolated and experimental arterial repairs, the routine practice of arterial reconstruction did not begin until the second half of the 20th century following the end of World War II. The leaders of our history committee realized that many of the pioneer surgeons of vascular disease who had actually invented or had been among the first to practice this type of surgery were still available in 2010 for interview. Furthermore, it was concluded that the opportunity to document a lasting record of this history was important—firsthand, in their own words.

There are several other histories which discuss vascular surgery in the 20th century as are outlined in Norman Rich's Foreword of this book. However, none of the others used video recording of detailed interviews as this one does. To hear the stories and the history directly from the participants, who you can see, is not only intriguing but lends a level of authenticity higher than if filtered through the hands of an historian. The current project, begun in 2011, is also uniquely valuable because such a large number of vascular surgeons have been interviewed. These videos are available now for easy viewing with this book, which channels the reader through the SVS website and onto YouTube.

The initial history project group included Calvin Ernst, Norman Rich, Roger Gregory, and James Yao, with Dr. Yao as the chairman. They selected "History Project Work Group" as the name for their committee and endeavor. These four founding members soon chose additional interviewers to help with the workload, including William Baker, Kenneth Cherry, Mark Eskandari, Melina

Kibbe, Peter Lawrence, Walter McCarthy, and Bill Pearce. Toward the last years of the project John (Jeb) Hallett, Richard Lynn and James Menzoian were invited to join.

The committee decided that the purpose of the project would be to record for posterity the thoughts of selected senior vascular surgeons. Embedded within the interviews would then be some of the history of vascular surgery itself, and also of the SVS. The intent was not to craft a complete text or history of these topics, but to leave a legacy of information in the words of some of the important participants. Just who to interview was initially perplexing. Obviously, all surgeons who had made their careers operating on arteries and were nearing retirement age around 2010 would possess a wealth of important and interesting perspectives related to the previous four or five decades of surgery. Eventually, the committee formulated the following selection criteria for individuals to be interviewed:

1. All individuals would be members of the SVS.
2. All past presidents of the SVS or the American Association for Vascular Surgery (also including past presidents of the former society, the International Society of Cardiovascular Surgery-North American chapter) would be included.
3. All those who had received a Lifetime Achievement Award or Innovation Award from the SVS would be included.
4. Honorary members of the SVS would be invited to be interviewed if they wished.
5. Specially selected interviewees would also be invited, including those who had contributed to the advancement of vascular surgery in an extraordinary way, surgeons with exceptional surgical experience, and surgeons who had been promoted to high administrative positions within their institutions.

Critical to the overall success of the project was James Yao's recruitment of the talented videographer and editor, Jan Muller. It was decided to only lightly edit the interviews to retain the personality and informality of the sessions. Almost all of the interviewees provided photographs of their careers, and sometimes of their families and childhoods, which Mr. Muller then included in the videos. It was decided that the individuals interviewed would have final jurisdiction over the content. In virtually every case they received the final video product to review for accuracy before it was made public on the SVS website. In some cases, changes were requested and edits were made.

The first interview was conducted by Roger Gregory, who interviewed Denton Cooley on September 26, 2011. The committee decided, as a general rule, to interview the oldest surgeons first. Many of the interviews were conducted at the American College of Surgeons building at 633 N. St. Clair St., Chicago, IL where the SVS previously had its headquarters on the 22nd floor. Others were conducted at the annual SVS meetings. A few were videoed at surgeon's homes or at their home university.

The interviews were all planned to be between 60 and 90 minutes in length. In each case, the interviewer prepared by studying the corresponding curriculum vitae, reading critical papers, presidential addresses and often discussing the individual with key associates. In many cases, the interviewee would be somewhat forewarned of the upcoming questions. The pace of conducting the interviews was fairly rapid with nine accomplished in 2011, 42 in 2012, 16 in 2013, eight in 2014, and five in 2015. There was one conducted in 2016, and the final two interviews, then totaling 83, were conducted on June 1, 2017 at the SVS national meeting in San Diego, California. To insure against any loss, two large, 6TB, backup hard drives were purchased to house all of the original and edited video and audio data that was otherwise stored on Mr. Muller's computer. These hard drives were placed at Dr. Yao and Dr. McCarthy's homes.

All of the video editing, including adding the still photographs provided by the interviewees, was conducted by James Yao and Jan Muller usually, at the Yaos' home. Along the way it was decided to add a written biography at the end of each video. The editing process and composing the biographies proved to be very time consuming—by December, 2017, only 14 of the interviews were completed and posted on the SVS website. At this point the history project committee had become sidetracked by many other interesting and important related endeavors. For example, Dr. Yao and Mr. Muller updated a detailed three-part history covering all of vascular surgery, which was produced with images in a DVD collection. The committee also traveled to Houston to visit the Michael DeBakey Museum, filming it and interviewing prominent surgeons there. Multiple national and international presentations were made with edited segments of the many interviews, including many two-minute "short segments" presented at SVS meetings. As time went by, the SVS executive committee notified the history project that there would not be any continued funding for the project. However, after a detailed presentation to the SVS by Dr. McCarthy, who had just around that time become chairman of the project, the SVS agreed to three additional years of funding to support Mr. Muller's editing efforts. This would allow the original project to be completed. However, it was formally stipulated, in writing, that no additional interviews or side projects should be conducted.

As the three-year funding deadline approached and Dr. Yao's health became a limiting factor, Dr. McCarthy and Mr. Muller completed the final 44 video postings in the last 18 months. The final posting was completed on June 8, 2022, just before the annual SVS meeting in Boston.

The original intent of the History Project Work Group had been to complete a great number of video interviews with prominent vascular surgeons to better document the history of the SVS and also the progress of vascular surgery itself over the last half century. Along the way, the concept of an accompanying book was proposed, initially envisioned as a collection of the transcripts from the interviews. Such a transcription collection book would have been thousands of pages long and seemed impractical. Therefore, the current book, a compendium, was envisioned linking biographies with the actual interviews using a QR code connection to the unique video URL YouTube address.

At the Boston meeting, Dr. McCarthy was able to explain to the SVS leadership the concept of a companion book, which would make the interviews more accessible, now that they were all on the SVS website. The committee was soon able to work through the logistics of "print on demand" through Amazon, using the publisher Amika Press of Northfield, Illinois, and an experienced editor, John Manos. The book would include a black-and-white photograph, a detailed biography and a QR code link to the YouTube video of each person. The videos are available in the history section of the SVS website, but having the QR code present would allow instant viewing by the reader on a smart phone. The copyright would be held by the SVS, which would be the recipient of the royalties. Writing the biographies either from scratch, or in many cases fact-checking and rewriting them, began in earnest in January, 2023 by Dr. McCarthy following Dr. Yao's sad death on December 20, 2022. Mr. Muller was of great assistance locating photographs, proofreading, fact checking, working on the QR codes and updating the video slides. John Manos, the editor, formatted and refined the writing.

Who should use this book

This book provides a guide to a vast and detailed slice of surgical history. It also, importantly, is a source for family members and friends to hear the voice and sense the significance of the interviewee within their chosen field, vascular surgery. In addition, surgeons who knew or trained with, or practice at the same institution as the interviewees, will be better able to understand their own surgical heritage by viewing the videos.

Vascular surgeons who wish to better navigate career avenues beyond clinical practice—including becoming hospital leaders, chiefs of vascular surgery, surgical department leaders, deans or medical center CEOs—will be able to hear from others who have done just that. Surgeons wishing to advance in academics and seeking strategies that are both intellectually rewarding and also successful will see pathways illustrated by many of the interviewees.

Surgeons or even historians interested in studying the development of arterial surgery, surgical technique, medical technology, prosthetic graft development, and medical device development will be able to watch interviews with people who did these things, and some who were even extremely successful as entrepreneurs. Historians interested in medical care during warfare, including detailed interviews of medical care from then-young surgeons who were in combat during World War II, the Korean War and the Vietnam War will find first-hand information from those who were there.

Individuals and historians interested in the history of the Society for Vascular Surgery, the *Journal of Vascular Surgery* and the development of the practice of vascular surgery as a specialty in the United States and around the world will find much original information. Those wanting to know more about medical publishing, successful textbook publication and the inner workings of surgical journals will not be disappointed. Finally, those seeking patterns for a successful professional life combined with a fulfilling personal and family life, including recreational pursuits, hobbies and even activity during retirement and guiding thoughts for people contemplating a surgical career will find inspiration and wisdom in many of the interviews.

LEGENDS
LEADERS
PIONEERS

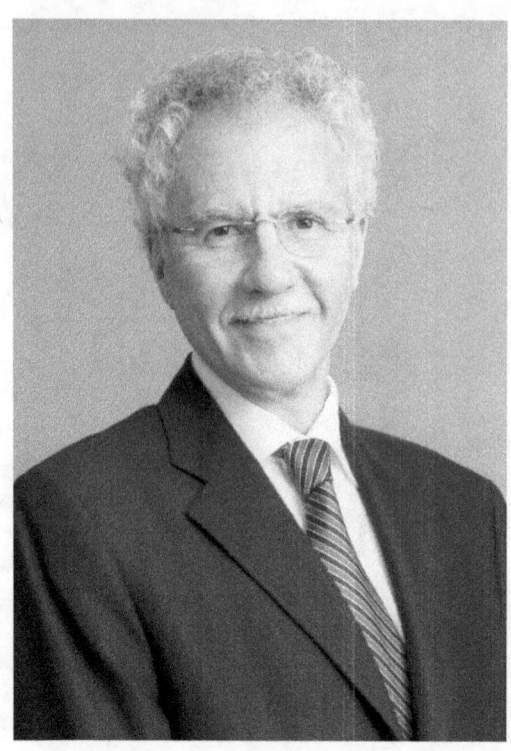

Enrico Ascher, MD

Enrico Ascher is a New York City vascular surgeon and surgical educator who completed his training in general surgery at New York Medical College. He then followed up with a one-year accredited vascular fellowship at Montefiore Medical Center and Albert Einstein Medical College in 1981–82. The program was directed by Frank Veith. Dr. Ascher stayed in the Bronx at Montefiore as a young attending where he continued to work with Dr. Veith and also with Dr. Henry Haimovici, both of whom he considers important surgical mentors.

After seven years at Montefiore, he moved to Brooklyn, New York to become the first board-certified vascular surgeon in Brooklyn. There he established a vascular surgery service and an accredited vascular surgery fellowship at Maimonides Medical Center, working there from 1983 until 2012. In 2012, he moved to NYU Langone Hospital in Brooklyn, becoming Chief of Vascular Surgery and establishing a vascular fellowship.

Besides his dedication to surgical training, Dr. Ascher has focused clinical research interests on lower extremity arterial disease and innovative ways to make open surgery and endovascular surgery less invasive. He has published more than 300 peer-reviewed articles in these areas. Academically, he has held appointments at five medical colleges in New York City, including attaining the rank of Professor of Surgery at Mount Sinai Medical School, which he has held since 2002.

Dr. Ascher's leadership skills have led him to the presidency of the Eastern Vascular Society, the Society for Clinical Vascular Surgery, the World Federation of Vascular Surgery, the International Society of Vascular Surgery and in 2006, the Society for Vascular Surgery.

Dr. Ascher has organized many national and international teaching meetings over the years including the important Pan-American Congress on Vascular Surgery which began in 1990 in Rio de Janeiro and meets every other year, bringing together surgeons of North and South America. He also organized the Vascular Fellows Abstract Competition that began in 1985, with an annual meeting held each year in New York City.

He was raised in Rio de Janeiro, Brazil, coming from a family in which all four children became physicians. He was born in Cairo, Egypt, where his father was in the petroleum business. The economy in Egypt changed when Gamel Nasser became president in 1954. The Ascher family, therefore, moved first to Europe and then permanently to Brazil when Dr. Ascher was six years old. He attended medical school at the Federal University of Rio de Janeiro, where he graduated in 1974. After a year of surgical training in Rio de Janeiro, he elected to move permanently to New York City for further training, where he remained for his entire distinguished surgical career.

Scan the QR code below or enter the YouTube link to watch the entire interview with Dr. Enrico Ascher conducted by Kenneth J. Cherry, MD, and James S.T. Yao, MD, brought to you by the SVS History Project Work Group.

 http://tinyurl.com/AscherXE

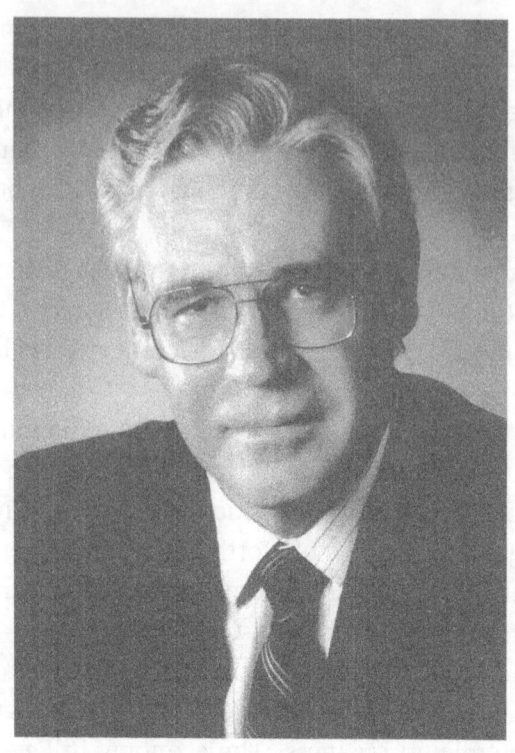

Ronald J. Baird, MD

Ronald Baird was a leading Canadian vascular and cardiac surgeon who trained under some of the great mid-20th century surgeons. Some of the legendary surgeons who guided him were Gordon Murray, Bill Bigelow and Bill Mustard in Toronto. Dr. Baird practiced during a time of incredible innovation in vascular surgery, with new devices and procedures. Beginning his career in the 1960s, he became an expert with a large practice in Toronto treating renal hypertension with endarterectomy and patch or using bypass. He performed many different operations for portal hypertension and was beginning his practice just as Dacron prostheses for aortic aneurysms were becoming available. By the 1970s, when saphenous vein aorto-coronary bypass became common, this and all types of open heart surgery also became an important part of Dr. Baird's practice. He performed the first human heart transplant in Toronto.

Dr. Baird became an authority on many historical developments such as the development of heparin. This was a special interest for him as his mentor,

Gordon Murray, had been the first surgeon to use heparin back in 1937. Dr. Baird was very involved in the organizational side of medicine and on one memorable occasion traveled to the Soviet Union for two months in 1960 to observe surgery and exchange ideas during the Cold War.

Born in 1930, Dr. Baird was the son of a Canadian railway porter and an American mother. His whole career was spent in Toronto, from his birth through his training and for the entirety of his practice. A 1954 graduate in medicine from the University of Toronto, he became a Professor of Surgery and Chairman of the Division of Cardiovascular Surgery at the University of Toronto, the Toronto Western Hospital and the Toronto General Hospital. He held Fellowships from the Royal College of Surgeons in Canada in general surgery and in cardiovascular surgery and thoracic surgery. He was awarded a Master of Surgery degree from the University of Toronto and the Medal in Surgery from the Royal College.

Dr. Baird was a past President of the North American Chapter of the International Society for Cardiovascular Surgery, the Canadian Cardiovascular Society, and the Canadian Society of Thoracic and Cardiovascular Surgeons. He was an honorary member of the Southern Society for Vascular Surgery, the American Association for Thoracic and Cardiovascular Surgery and the Society for Vascular Surgery.

During his distinguished career he wrote extensively on surgery of the heart and the arteries, and he developed several new procedures in both fields of surgery. He was proud to have trained over 60 surgeons.

Dr. Baird died of pneumonia on March 26, 2017 in Fort Lauderdale, Florida.

Scan the QR code below or enter the YouTube link to watch the entire interview with Dr. Ronald J. Baird conducted by Walter J. McCarthy, MD, brought to you by the SVS History Project Work Group.

 http://tinyurl.com/BairdXR1

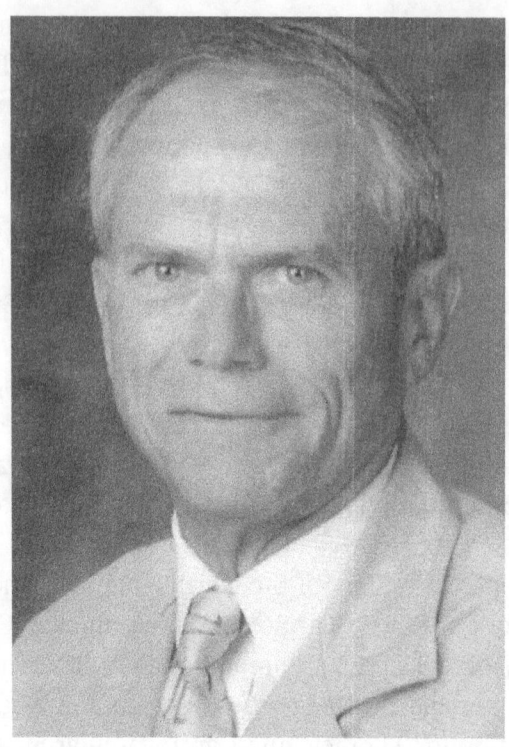

William H. Baker, MD

William H. Baker was born and raised on the south side of Chicago. His physician parents both practiced in the city, his father in urology and his mother in obstetrics and gynecology. Dr. Baker attended Chicago public schools, Knox College in Galesburg, Illinois, and the University of Chicago School of Medicine, graduating in the class of 1962.

His University of Chicago surgical internship was followed by a year in surgical residency at the University of Iowa Hospitals. He then spent two years in the Army at Fort Lawton in Seattle, Washington, and overseas with the 85th Evacuation Hospital in Viet Nam. He returned to Chicago to complete a general surgical residency at the University of Chicago Hospitals. He was then able to enroll in a fellowship in vascular surgery at the University of California San Francisco with Jack Wylie, W.K. Ehrenfeld and Ronald J. Stoney in 1969–1970.

Dr. Baker then joined the surgical faculty at the University of Iowa where he established a vascular service and fellowship. In 1976, he was recruited to the faculty at Loyola University of Chicago, where he remained for the rest of his distinguished career. At Loyola, he was the Chief of Peripheral Vascular Surgery, the program director of both general surgery and the vascular surgery fellowship and Director of the Peripheral Vascular Diagnostic Laboratory.

Dr. Baker is an author of approximately 150 articles and 60 book chapters. He is perhaps best known for his carotid endarterectomy-related surgical contributions and publications. He was the President of the Association of Vascular Surgery Program Directors, the North American Chapter of the ISCVS, the Midwestern Vascular Surgical Society, the Central Surgical Association, the Midwest Surgical Association and the Chicago Surgical Society. He is particularly proud of the expertise of the Loyola Vascular Section and of the accomplishments of the Loyola vascular fellows.

In retirement, Dr. Baker plays golf, a little tennis, and bicycles. His four granddaughters live in Oak Park, and he and his wife, Ann, enjoy them immensely, both in Oak Park and at their home in Michigan. He continues to teach, tutoring grade-schoolers in Chicago two mornings a week, and attends the vascular conference at Loyola.

Scan the QR code below or enter the YouTube link to watch the entire interview with Dr. William H. Baker conducted by Walter J. McCarthy, MD, brought to you by the SVS History Project Work Group.

 http://tinyurl.com/BakerXW

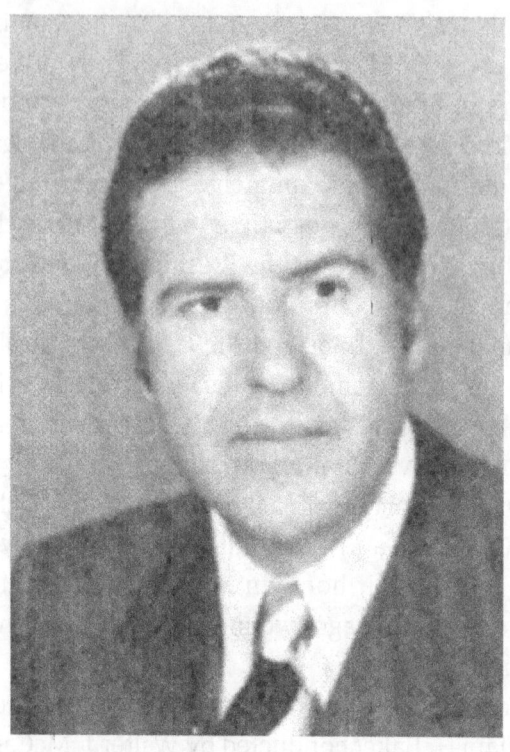

Panagiotis E. Balas, MD

One could say that Panagiotis Balas' career, like so many surgeons of his generation, was very much shaped by his early contact with Dr. Michael DeBakey in Houston. Born and trained in Greece, he arrived in Houston for a clinical fellowship in 1960. He was very impressed by Dr. DeBakey's mission to train surgeons from all over the world. Dr. Balas followed Dr. DeBakey's example by introducing vascular surgery to Greece and by hosting many international meetings there. He made many visits to China and Russia and made a personal effort to encourage surgeons to visit the West for conferences and training. Years later, in 1977, he presented his mentor, Dr. Debakey, with a sculpture of one of Dr. DeBakey's hands crafted by a Greek sculptor. Dr. Balas commented, "You always said if you had a third hand, you could get more accomplished."

Dr. Panagiotis ("Taki") Balas was born in Kalamata, Greece, but grew up in Athens. Both his father and his uncle were physicians. He graduated from medical school in 1953 and began an internship in general surgery. He worked at the first surgical clinic in Greece at the Athens University Medical School under Dr. Nicolas Christeas. Dr. Christeas had been a student of Dr. René Leriche in Strasbourg in 1938 at the same time that Dr. Michael DeBakey studied there.

Following six years in Athens, Dr. Balas took a research fellowship at the New England Medical Center under Dr. Allan Callow, earning an MS in Surgery. In 1960, he was appointed to a clinical fellowship in Houston under Dr. Michael DeBakey, where he stayed for three years.

Upon his return to Greece in 1963, Dr. Balas began introducing modern vascular surgery to his home country. He performed many vascular surgical firsts in Greece. He also developed an audio-visual department that captured his work on color movie film. Dr. Balas is very well known for his work in microvascular surgery, specifically for a procedure in which he saved an amputated finger. He also performed the first reimplantation of a completely amputated upper extremity.

Dr. Balas began work as a meeting organizer in 1966 when he founded the Michael DeBakey Society, an annual international congress. He continued these efforts by hosting the International Union of Angiology (IUA) Congress in 1980 in Athens, as well as the International Society for Cardiovascular Surgery meeting in 1981. While hosting the IUA Congress, Dr. Balas served as its president. During his term, he shifted the organization from a primarily French group to a more inclusive, international body, changing its constitution and its main language to English for both the subsequent meetings and for its journal.

The theme of international exchange was the driving force behind Dr. Balas' writing. In articles, he featured the influence of European vascular surgeons on North American vascular surgery and the returned influence of American surgery on European practice by the many surgeons who were trained in the U.S.

To advance technological changes in vascular surgery, Dr. Balas participated in the founding of the International Endovascular Society in 1993 with Dr. Ted Diethrich. Soon afterwards, Dr. Balas performed the first endovascular treatment for abdominal aortic aneurysm in Greece in 1996. Among his many honors he was inducted as an Honorary Fellow of the American College of Surgeons in 1993.

Scan the QR code below or enter the YouTube link to watch the entire interview with Dr. Panagiotis E. Balas conducted by Norman M. Rich, MD, and James S.T. Yao, MD, brought to you by the SVS History Project Work Group.

 http://tinyurl.com/BalasXP

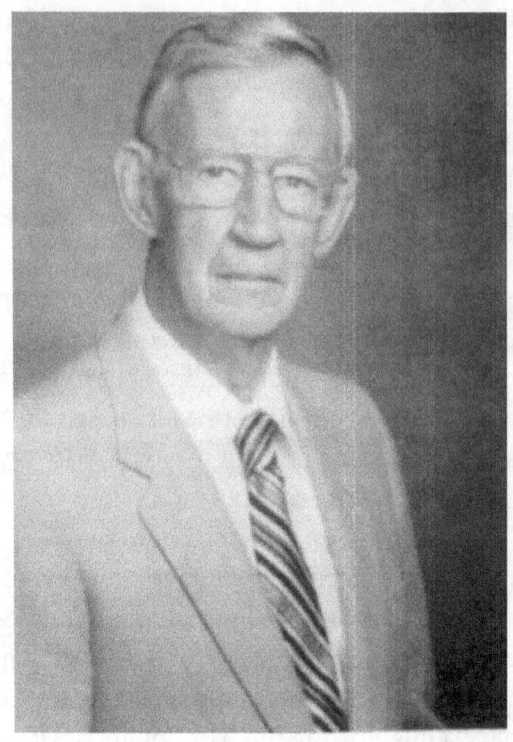

Wylie F. Barker, MD

Wylie Franklin Barker was born in Santa Fe, New Mexico, on October 16, 1919. His New Mexico roots were deep, with family in the region since long before statehood—his grandfather established a ranch there in 1888.

Dr. Barker received his bachelor and medical degrees from Harvard University. This education was followed by 18 months of residency at the Peter Bent Brigham Hospital in Boston under Dr. Elliot Cutler. He enlisted in the United States Navy, first serving six months of very active surgical duty at the Chelsea Naval Hospital in Boston, Massachusetts, and then aboard the *USS Grand Canyon*, a Navy destroyer tender headquartered in Naples, Italy, in 1946. This was followed by six months at Portsmouth Naval Hospital in Norfolk, Virginia.

He returned to the Brigham in 1947 for another 18 months of training during which he worked under the pioneer vascular surgeon John Homans. Dr. Barker then traveled west to Los Angeles in 1949 to assist Dr. William P. Longmire in forming a full-time university surgical department at the new UCLA

Medical Center. There he became Professor and Chief of General Surgery and the Director of the Peripheral Vascular service. He also served as the Chief of Staff of the Sepulveda VA Hospital from 1978 to 1983.

Among Dr. Barker's many publications, his textbook, *Surgical Treatment of Peripheral Vascular Disease,* was one of the most highly recognized. He is remembered for having developed a device for remote arterial endarterectomy with his colleague Jack Cannon. The instrument, a ring stripper which they fabricated from piano wire, allowed the removal of long segments of atherosclerosis from the superficial femoral artery through short incisions. Dr. Barker served as President of the Society for Vascular Surgery in 1973, and he remained at UCLA—where an endowed Chair has been established in his name—until his retirement in 1986.

Dr. Barker and his wife Nancy raised three children: Robert, Jonathan and Christina. Dr. Barker's special medical interests included peripheral vascular disease, diseases of the breast and inflammatory bowel problems. In retirement Dr. Barker enjoyed orchid culture, sold orchids and authored a book on that subject. A capable horseback rider since his New Mexico boyhood, he completed many seven- to ten-day high wilderness horseback trail rides throughout the Rocky Mountains.

Dr. Barker died at the age of 94 on October 31, 2013.

Scan the QR code below or enter the YouTube link to watch the entire interview with Dr. Wylie F. Barker conducted by Peter F. Lawrence, MD, brought to you by the SVS History Project Work Group.

 http://tinyurl.com/BarkerXW

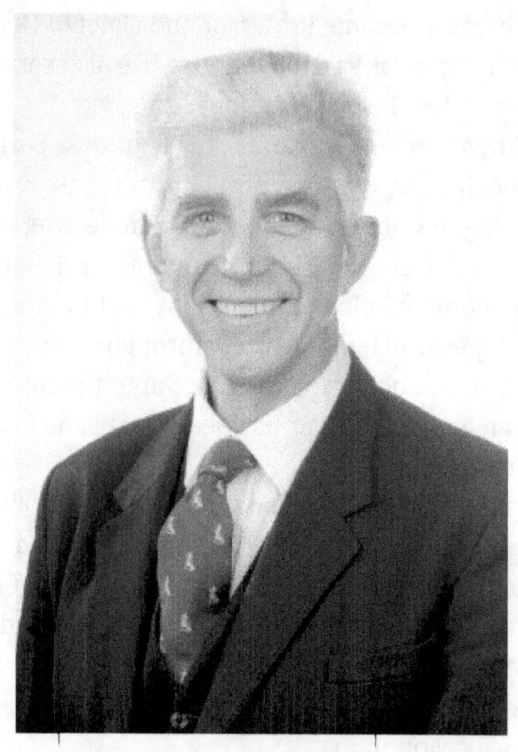

Jonathan D. Beard, MD

Jonathan Beard was born and raised in the southeast of England in Chelmsford, Essex. His father, John, was an electronic engineer and although Jonathan had a keen interest in electronics as a child, his father persuaded him to pursue a career in medicine.

He trained at Guy's Hospital in London where he also played rugby. During his time at Guy's, Mr. Beard undertook an intercalcated BSc in physics applied to medicine and wrote a dissertation on fast Fourier transform analysis of blood flow waveforms. After qualifying as MB BS (Guy's Hospital, London) in 1979, he worked as an anatomy demonstrator at the Middlesex Hospital and became a Fellow of the Royal College of Surgeons of England.

During his training he was inspired by Mr. John Fairgreive, one of the original vascular surgeons in England. He subsequently was trained under the supervision of Professor Michael Horrocks and later worked under Professor Sir Peter Bell. Through these mentors he became involved with the European

Society for Vascular Surgery, and became interested in surgical writing. After working with the *European Journal of Vascular and Endovascular Surgery* for nearly 20 years, he was appointed as Editor-in-Chief in 2005.

Mr. Beard was appointed as the first full-time vascular surgeon to the Sheffield Teaching Hospitals in 1990 where he helped form one of the first citywide vascular units in the country to offer 24/7 emergency vascular care.

He has a lifetime research interest in electronics and Doppler analysis of vascular problems and an interest in contributing patients to and directing vascular trials. His special interest in surgical education inspired him to obtain a master's degree in this area from the University of Sheffield. Clinically he has a passionate interest in amputation techniques, quality-of-life outcomes and also exercise therapy for intermittent claudication.

Professor Beard served as the President of the Vascular Society of Great Britain and Ireland in 2014 and as Professor of Surgical Education at the Royal College. In 1998 Professor Beard published, with his co-author Peter Gaines, a highly respected textbook, *Vascular and Endovascular Surgery*. The book is now in its 6th edition.

Professor Beard is married with two sons and his leisure interests include rugby, downhill skiing with his wife and children, road cycling, sailing his catamaran and singing barbershop.

Scan the QR code below or enter the YouTube link to watch the entire interview with Professor Jonathan D. Beard conducted by Roger T. Gregory, MD, brought to you by the SVS History Project Work Group.

 http://tinyurl.com/BeardXJ

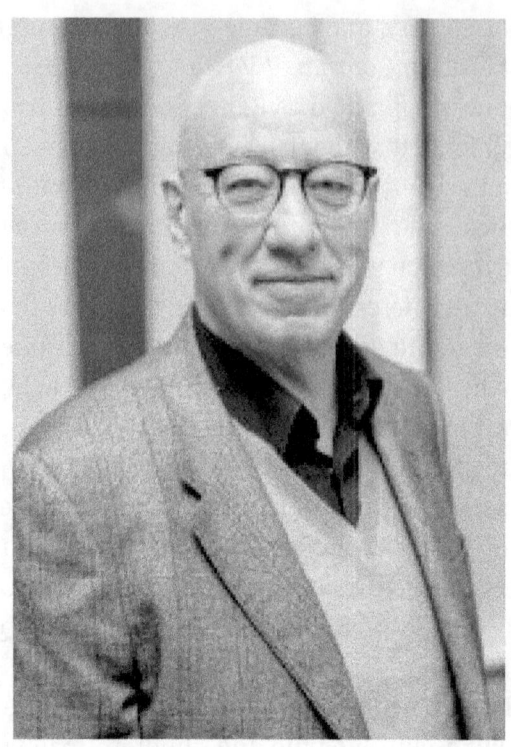

Jean-Pierre Becquemin, MD

Jean-Pierre Becquemin is an International Member of the Society for Vascular Surgery and serves as Professor of Vascular Surgery at the Henri Mandor Hospital in Paris. He has been the Section Head there since November 16, 2005. His hospital is located in Creteil, France, which is just outside of central Paris. Dr. Becquemin has experience in all areas of vascular surgery, but he has a particular interest in endovascular aortic aneurysm surgery, including endovascular treatment of ruptured aortic aneurysms. He has developed a center to manage acute vascular problems including pre- and post-operative care, imaging, anesthesia and operative intervention. He was an early adopter of endovascular aortic repair for both the abdominal and thoracic aorta, as well as endovascular intervention of more peripheral lesions including carotid arteries. He began using endovascular aortic repair in 1994 in France and soon afterward traveled to Australia to spend six months in Sidney with Jim May. Dr. May assured him that "endo" was indeed the future of aortic surgery.

Dr. Becquemin was raised in Fontainebleau, a town 40 miles southeast of Paris, where he also went to college. Fontainebleau is known for its hiking and rock climbing, and Jean-Pierre was drawn to these endeavors at a young age. College was followed by medical school in Paris. The young Dr. Becquemin was inspired by the pioneering work of Jacques Oudot, also a mountain climber, who many years before had been the first to operate on the occluded abdominal aorta.

During his training, Dr. Becquemin worked directly under Charles Dubost, who had performed the first successful aortic aneurysm repair with an implanted graft. This was done using a homograft on March 29, 1951. Dubost, by then a very senior surgeon in the late 1970s, advised and persuaded his young trainee that vascular surgery would be a great career.

Dr. Becquemin is the Chairman and creator of an important international meeting and educational program entitled "Controversies and Updates in Vascular Surgery." The 25th session of this well-known course was held January 23–25, 2020 in Paris, France. Sixty countries were represented with well over 1000 registrants during the three-day conference.

Among his many awards, Dr. Becquemin has been honored as a Fellow of the Royal College of Surgeons.

Scan the QR code below or enter the YouTube link to watch the entire interview with Dr. Jean-Pierre Becquemin conducted by Walter J. McCarthy, MD, and James S.T. Yao, MD, brought to you by the SVS History Project Work Group.

 http://tinyurl.com/BecquXJP

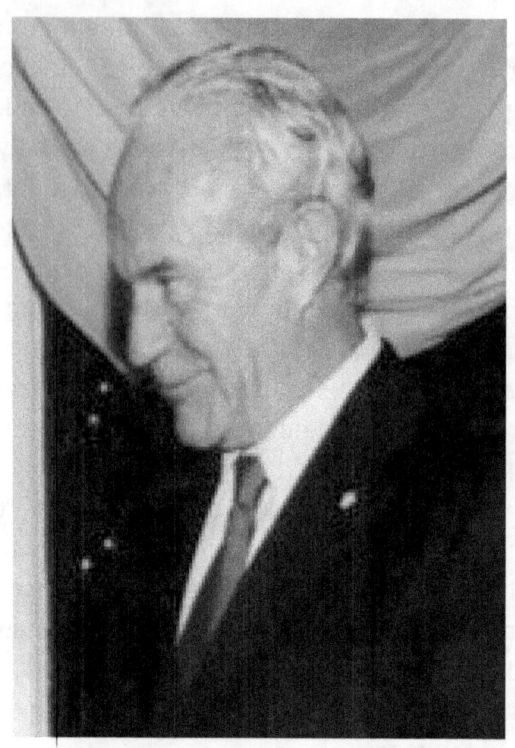

Ramon Berguer, MD, PhD

Ramon Berguer, President of the Society for Vascular Surgery from 2000 to 2001, is a multi-talented individual. Not only is he a distinguished academic surgeon, he is also a formula car racer, a PhD in Engineering from the University of Surrey, England, and also avid in his pursuit of a lifelong interest in art, mathematics and philosophy. One of the unique features of the *Annals of Vascular Surgery,* which Dr. Berguer founded, is the artwork featured on the cover of each issue, which he selects and accompanies with a brief description.

Ramon Berguer was born in Barcelona, Spain. His family experienced both the Spanish Civil War and World War II and was exposed to the suffering of food rationing. His father was a dentist, and his mother was a teacher. His grandfather was a surgeon. Dr. Bergeur went to college in Spain and in 1962 received an MD degree from the University of Barcelona. Completing medical school, he was accepted into an internship program at the University of Santiago Medical School in Spain. Then, after two years of military service, he traveled to America for additional medical training. He began another internship at Washington Hospital Center in Washington, DC. Following his internship, he scheduled an interview with Dr. Emerick Szilagyi and was accepted to Henry Ford Hospital in Detroit for residency training in general and vascular surgery. During this period, he developed an interest in bioengineering. While he was a surgical resident at Henry Ford, Dr. Szilagyi arranged for him to spend a year studying mathematics in Detroit.

Following his surgical training in Detroit, he returned to Spain and became involved in the organization of resistance against the dictator General Franco. Within a year he needed to leave Spain to avoid detention and in 1972 departed for London. He pursued further training in the Department of Biomedical Engineering, King's College, University of London, and also within the Department of Surgery. In 1974, due to the difficulty of career advancement in England, he returned to the United States. On the advice of his mentor, Dr. Szilagyi, he accepted the position of Assistant Professor of Surgery at Wayne State University Medical School in Detroit.

Under the direction of Dr. Berguer, Wayne State University emerged as a center of excellence in vascular surgery. Dr. Berguer has made multiple contributions to vascular surgery. He is known for his interest in cerebral ischemia and developed and became the director of the first stroke unit at Wayne. The stroke unit combined expert care from vascular surgery, cardiology and interventional radiology. A unique focus of Dr. Berguer's career has been surgery of the vertebral artery. His contribution in this area is unparalleled, involving reconstruction not only at the vertebral artery's origin but also with extensive experience in the C-1, C-2 location. His textbook, *Surgery of the Arteries of the Head*, co-authored with Edouard Kieffer, is a classic.

Leaving Wayne State University after 30 years, he moved to the University of Michigan in 2004, where he was named the Frankel Professor of Surgery. There he has continued his study of aortic hemodynamics, especially the effect of the endovascular graft by using mechanical and mathematical modeling.

Recently, Dr. Berguer has purchased and restored seaside property in northwest Spain. In this area of his youth, Galicia, he has taken up viticulture, growing grapes in his own vineyard.

Scan the QR code below or enter the YouTube link to watch the entire interview with Dr. Ramon Berguer conducted by William H. Baker, MD, brought to you by the SVS History Project Work Group.

 http://tinyurl.com/BerguerXR

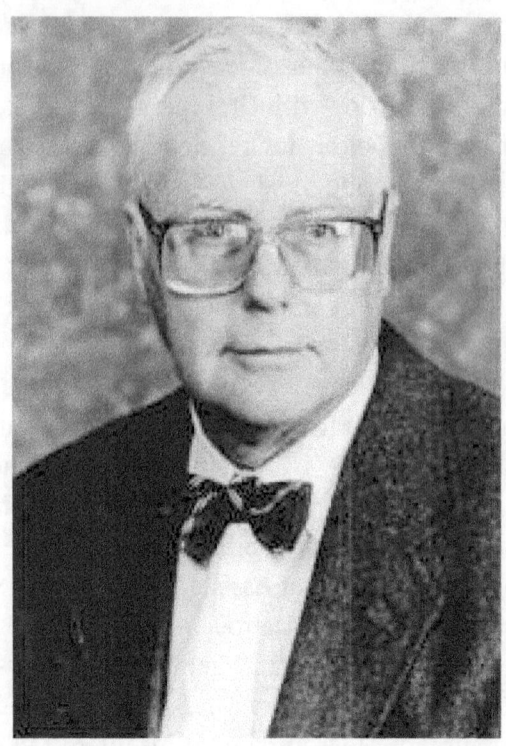

F. William Blaisdell, MD

The renowned surgeon Bill Blaisdell was born and raised in California and practiced there his entire life. He was born in Santa Barbara and moved to Watsonville at age five. He grew up in an agricultural community where his father, an internist, was in practice with Bill's uncle, who was a general surgeon. Both of Bill's grandfathers were doctors, and virtually all of the other members of his family were as well.

Two past generations had attended Stanford University, and that is where Dr. Blaisdell completed college, medical school and general surgical training. During surgical residency, he spent one year in Boston with Dr. Frances "Frannie" Moore and was thereby introduced to surgical research, which he pursued throughout his entire career. An important surgical mentor, Richard Warren, told him that if he wanted to be a vascular surgeon, he should go to Houston to train with Michael DeBakey, which he did. He was there for one year, which also included training under Denton Cooley and Stanley Crawford. He credits his experience in Houston with giving him the idea of axillary femoral-femoral bypass, which he invented and was the first to perform. His idea was to use the "ax-fem" as a back-up operation for lower extremity arterial reconstruction.

He returned from Houston to San Francisco in 1960, was appointed the Chief of Surgery at the San Francisco VA, and then in 1966, he became the Chief of Surgery at San Francisco General Hospital. There he set up the very first comprehensive city-wide trauma unit in the United States and thereafter became one of the most experienced surgical trauma experts in the country. He practiced vascular, trauma and cardiac surgery.

In 1978, Dr. Blaisdell was recruited to be the Chief of Surgery at the University of California, Davis, in Sacramento. He developed that program into a fine surgical unit. When he retired in 1995, as a tribute to his dedication to teaching at the university, the new medical library at the UC Davis was named the F. William Blaisdell Library.

Dr. Blaisdell published more than 321 papers and book chapters and many books, particularly on trauma surgery. Besides inventing the axillary femoral-femoral bypass, he also was the first to report a descending thoracic aorta to femoral bypass operation. He did some of the very first research on what is now called ARDS. He became interested in the control of bleeding and the use of heparin early in his career and published much in that area. He served as the President of the Society for Vascular Surgery from 1978–1979 and was President of the American Association for the Surgery of Trauma among his many other prestigious accomplishments.

As a young man Dr. Blaisdell was married to his wife Marilyn, with whom he had six children, and who preceded him in death by several years. Dr. Blaisdell is remembered as a gentleman and for his energy, intelligence, and for his "niceness." He pursued hobbies including the history of railroads, the Civil War, Civil War medicine, magic, model airplanes, and tennis. He also wrote mystery novels. He died on April 18, 2020.

Scan the QR code below or enter the YouTube link to watch the entire interview with Dr. F. William Blaisdell conducted by Norman M. Rich, MD, brought to you by the SVS History Project Work Group.

 http://tinyurl.com/BlaisdellXW

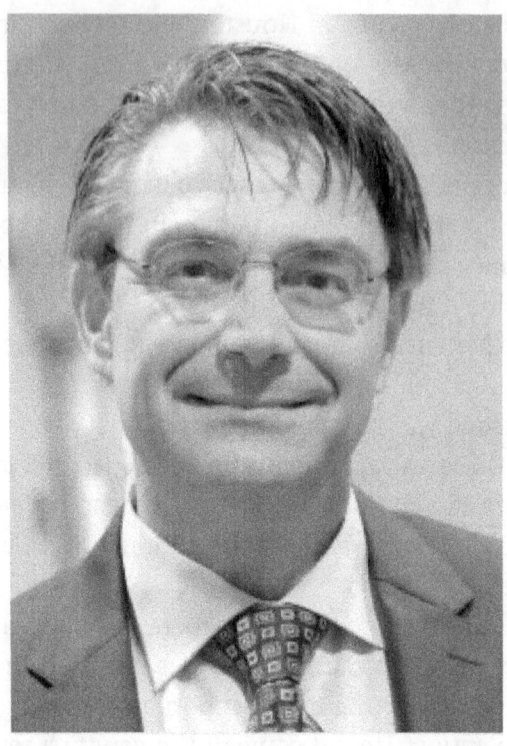

Jan D. Blankensteijn, MD, PhD

Jan D. Blankensteijn was born in Oranjestad, Aruba, in the Dutch Antilles in 1959. When he was very young, his family moved to the south of the Netherlands where he was raised. He knew as early as age eleven that he wanted to go into medicine, since he was fascinated with surgery. He attended medical school at the University of Utrecht from 1977–1984. In the mid-1980s in the Netherlands, there were too many surgeons for the available positions. Programs accepted as few as 16 residents per year nationwide. Fortunately, Dr. Blankensteijn was accepted into several residencies throughout the Netherlands, and he selected Erasmus University in Rotterdam.

Upon finishing this training in 1992, he started a fellowship in liver transplantation which evolved into a PhD thesis at Erasmus University.

Because of a close link between the Netherlands and the Massachusetts General Hospital in Boston, Dr. Blankensteijn was able to travel there for a one-year Associate Clinical Fellowship under Dr. William Abbott. During his exit interview, Dr. Abbott showed him an issue of the *Journal of Vascular Surgery* that featured an advertisement for a new technique for percutaneous aneurysm repair. The term endovascular had yet to be coined.

With his certificate from the Mass General, Dr. Blankensteijn returned to the Netherlands to be the vascular surgery fellow in Rotterdam. Vascular surgery was still a sub-specialty of general surgery at the time. In 1994, Dr. Blankensteijn was offered a position at the University Medical Center in Utrecht, leading a percutaneous surgery program with the early Endovascular Technology (EVT) endovascular aortic grafting equipment. In 1994, he performed the first endovascular procedure in Utrecht after a trip to Los Angeles to observe the technique as performed by Dr. Wesley Moore.

In 1994, Dr. Blankensteijn began writing grants for research, making comparisons between open and endovascular aortic results, which were initially delayed because of early complications with the new procedure. Finally, in 1999, with him serving as the principal investigator, the Dutch Randomized Endovascular Aneurysm Management (DREAM) Trial began.

Dr. Blankensteijn has more than 200 publications with over 11,000 citations many related to aortic aneurysm surgery and the DREAM Trial. Dr. Blakensteijn has been a Professor of Vascular Surgery at the VU Medical Center in Amsterdam since 2009.

Scan the QR code below or enter the YouTube link to watch the entire interview with Dr. Jan D. Blankensteijn conducted by Walter J. McCarthy, MD, and James S.T. Yao, MD, brought to you by the SVS History Project Work Group.

 http://tinyurl.com/BlankXJ1

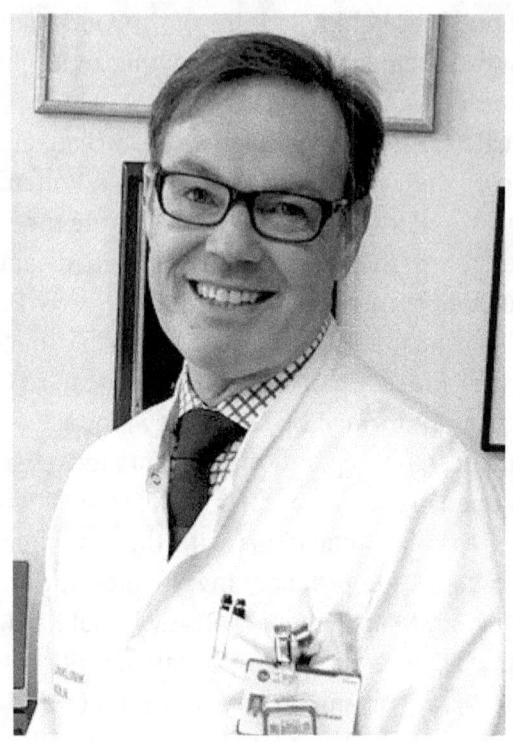

Jan S. Brunkwall, MD

Jan S. Brunkwall was born in Stockholm, Sweden, where his mother was a nurse and his father a veterinary student. When he was just a few years old, his family moved to the south of Sweden, where his father took a position as a veterinarian. He began his schooling there, finishing high school in 1972, near the Danish border. He always knew he wanted to go into medicine since he had assisted his father in his veterinary practice from a very young age. At the age of twelve, due to the influence of a family friend who was a general practitioner, he became interested in working with patients with whom he could better communicate!

Dr. Brunkwall applied to Lund University, which was very competitive. He took time off to study French in case he had to attend his second-choice school in Leuven, Belgium. However, he was accepted to Lund and decided during his first year that he would be a vascular surgeon. After five and one-half years in Lund, Dr. Brunkwall transferred to Halmstad, north of Malmö where he could obtain more surgical experience. He stayed there for five years in a general surgery residency, focusing on vascular surgery because of the excellent program in Halmstad.

From 1986–87, after an invitation from Dr. James Stanley, Dr. Brunkwall traveled to Ann Arbor, Michigan, to do research and clinical work. His subsequent work on prostanoid vessel wall release eventually led to a PhD thesis in 1990. His paper was published in the *European Journal of Vascular Surgery*. He then returned to Malmö to continue research. Shortly after his return, the Chief of General Surgery in Cologne, Germany, contacted him about a position there. Dr. Brunkwall and his wife, who is German, then accepted an appointment as an associate professor to establish a vascular surgery practice in Cologne. After 13 years, Dr. Brunkwall gradually tripled the size of the Cologne unit and expanded the range of procedures offered.

Dr. Brunkwall is an Honorary Member of the Society for Vascular Surgery. After years spent training and practicing in numerous countries, Dr. Brunkwall is able to offer many comparisons between surgical practice in the U.S. and Europe.

Scan the QR code below or enter the YouTube link to watch the entire interview with Dr. Jan S. Brunkwall conducted by Norman M. Rich, MD, brought to you by the SVS History Project Work Group.

 http://tinyurl.com/BrunkwallXJ

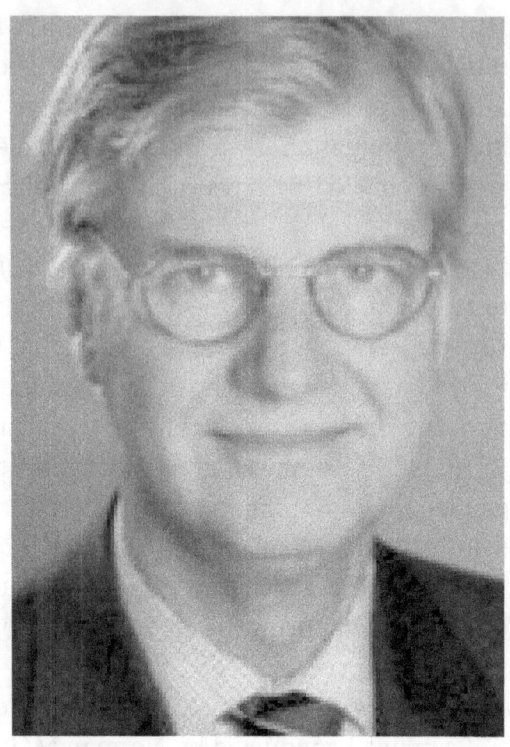

Jacob Buth, MD

Jacob "Jaap" Buth, formerly consulting vascular surgeon and Chief of Vascular Surgery in Eindhoven, the Netherlands, was born on January 22, 1944, in the village of Den Bommel, on the isle of Goeree-Overflakkee in the southwest of the Netherlands. He spent his childhood and high school years in that area. His father had been a general practitioner on the island from the beginning of World War II. His mother came from the same region. Jacob had considered going into engineering and shipbuilding, but chose medicine realizing that the shipbuilding industry was then being outsourced to the developing world.

On his 17th birthday, he therefore traveled to Utrecht University to study medicine, which was the same school that his father had attended. He graduated in 1966 and relocated to Rotterdam for an internship at the University and its affiliated hospitals.

Dr. Buth's surgical training started in 1970 in Rotterdam under professor Piet Kooreman and later under Dr. Gerard Olthuis as the Chiefs of Staff. In

1974 and 1975, he was accepted into a clinical fellowship at the Massachusetts General Hospital (MGH) with Dr. R. Clement Darling, Jr. Interestingly, he had been initially attracted to vascular surgery as a specialty by the articles he had read by Dr. Darling.

After returning from Boston, he finished surgical training and graduated with a PhD in 1978 under Professor Reinier van Dongen at Amsterdam University. The title of his thesis was *The Vascular Laboratory*. His analysis was based on clinical and physiologic data collected at the MGH. In 1979, he moved to the Catharina Hospital, a large teaching hospital in Eindhoven. His practice started with mostly general surgery; however, it was soon dedicated to vascular surgery, including an active teaching program.

Some of Dr. Buth's accomplishments include: Executive Director of EUROSTAR, an International Collaborative Registry of data of Endovascular Abdominal Aortic Repair and Thoracic Endovascular Aortic Repair, 1996–2007; President of the Dutch Society of Vascular Surgery; Secretary of the European Board of Vascular Surgery at the UEMS (Union Européenne des Médecins Spécialistes); Associate Editor of the *European Journal of Vascular and Endovascular Surgery* (EJVES); and editorial board member of the *Journal of Vascular Surgery*. Dr. Buth's current positions include Consulting Vascular Surgeon Da Vinci Clinic-Geldrop; Editorial Board member of the EJVES; and Honorary member of the SVS. Dr. Buth's clinical research includes more than 150 peer-reviewed publications and 150 non-peer reviewed publications and book chapters.

Scan the QR code below or enter the YouTube link to watch the entire interview with Dr. Jacob Buth conducted by Roger T. Gregory, MD, and James S.T. Yao, MD, brought to you by the SVS History Project Work Group.

 http://tinyurl.com/ButhXJ

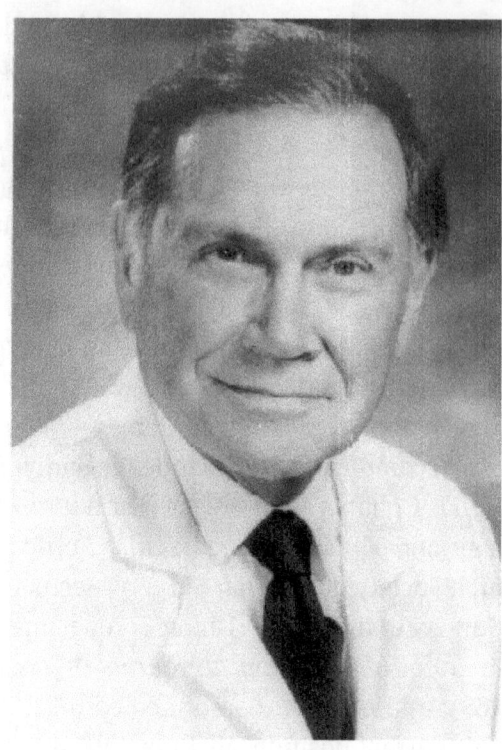

Allan D. Callow, MD

Allan Callow's family moved from Scotland to Maine by way of Liverpool and the Isle of Man in 1628. They changed the family name from McCullough to Callow along the way. Dr. Callow was the first physician from a family who had been farmers, fishermen, carpenters and who also had worked in the shipping and railroad industries.

His high school French teacher was an early mentor encouraging him to become a plant geneticist. He earned a BS degree from Tufts University in 1938. Dr. Callow then went on to Harvard Medical School, which he found to be full of hard work, but was overall "a romp." He graduated in 1942 and began an internship at the Massachusetts General and Peter Bent Brigham Hospitals.

In 1939 Dr. Callow had secured a naval reserve commission, which he pursued because of his family's maritime experience, and he became a voluntary probationary ensign in the U.S. Navy in 1939. With World War II raging, Dr. Callow was assigned to the *USS Henry Lee* in 1943. His unit trained on the west coast to be a beach-landing battalion in the Pacific Theater. Dr. Callow participated as a medical officer in seven major landing parties under heavy fire. He said that living through a bombardment taught him to discard what was trivial. He developed a tremendous respect for the persistence of the ordinary soldier, which later led him to write *The Man on the Ground: Who Really Wins Our Wars?* in 2013. Dr. Callow was eventually promoted to Rear Admiral, and he served in that capacity from 1968 through 1978.

After WWII, he worked as a research assistant for three years and earned a PhD. Later, during his surgical training, he selected the specialty of vascular surgery because of his wartime experience. Dr. Callow was frustrated by how many young lives were diminished by amputations that could have been avoided had vascular repair been available. This same spirit propelled him into carotid surgery in the early 1950s to try to address the problem of stroke. After hundreds of cases, he learned to carefully select patients, and this led to sustained success. He published *Surgery of the Carotid and Vertebral Arteries for the Prevention of Stroke* in 1996.

On the organizational side of medicine, Dr. Callow was an advocate for research funding, spearheading the creation of the Lifeline Foundation 501(c)(3) within the SVS. This foundation has subsequently awarded hundreds of student fellowships, dozens of Wiley Travelling Fellowships and dozens of K08 and K23 grants. Later in his career he returned to Tufts University, first as a Trustee and then as Chairman of the Board, where he greatly transformed the institution. He served as President of the ISCVS-NA in 1975 and of the SVS in 1986.

In his 70s, Dr. Callow married the dynamic biomedical researcher Dr. Una Ryan. At age 99 he died at home in San Francisco with her by his side on December 22, 2015.

Scan the QR code below or enter the YouTube link to watch the entire interview with Dr. Allan D. Callow conducted by Norman M. Rich, MD, brought to you by the SVS History Project Work Group.

 http://tinyurl.com/CallowXA

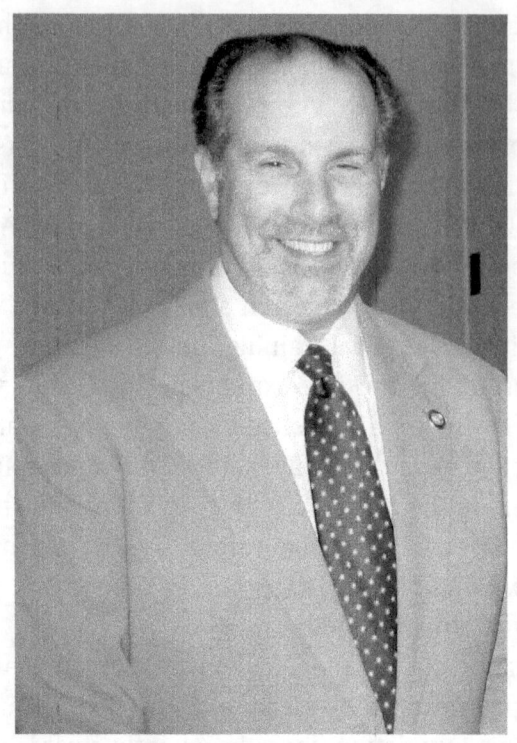

Richard P. Cambria, MD

Richard P. Cambria is a Boston surgeon who was born on May 18, 1951, in Elizabeth, NJ. He attended college at Holy Cross and had the fortunate career-shaping opportunity to work as a surgical technician during college summer breaks. His subsequent education involved completing medical school at Columbia University which included some intriguing exposure to vascular surgery. As a medical student at Columbia, he remembers, one Saturday morning scrubbing in on a case with Arthur Voorhees. Dr. Voorhees was the first surgeon to have implanted a synthetic fabric vascular graft in a human aorta, which he had done years before, in 1953.

However, the majority of Dr. Cambria's surgical training was at the Massachusetts General Hospital, beginning with a sub-internship in 1976 with R. Clement Darling, Jr. His rotation with Dr. Darling convinced him that he wanted to become a vascular surgeon. Surgical residency and formal vascular training followed at Massachusetts General. There he was the first Robert R.

Linton Vascular Research Fellow and worked in the laboratory with William Abbott, who was the Chief of Vascular Surgery at that time. It is of interest that years later in 2012, Dr. Cambria became the inaugural Robert R. Linton Professor of Vascular and Endovascular Surgery at the Harvard University Medical School.

Dr. Cambria's first appointment as a surgical attending was at Yale in 1985, but he soon returned to the Massachusetts General Hospital and eventually became the Chief of Vascular and Endovascular Surgery (2002–2017) and the Program Director of the Vascular Fellowship (2002–2008). Since 2017, he has been the Chief of Vascular and Endovascular Surgery at Saint Elizabeth's Hospital in Boston.

Dr. Cambria has had a major research and clinical career interest in vascular surgery for complex aortic disease, including both the abdominal and the thoracic aorta. His original thinking about this topic and very extensive case volume have positioned him as a world expert in this type of surgery. He has had a particular interest in the vexing problem of spinal cord ischemia after thoracoabdominal aneurysm surgery. Many of his most important contributions are in this area.

Dr. Cambria's leadership skills have led to his Presidency of the New England Society for Vascular Surgery (2008–2009) and the Society for Vascular Surgery (2011–2012).

Scan the QR code below or enter the YouTube link to watch the entire interview with Dr. Richard P. Cambria conducted by William H. Pearce, MD, and William H. Baker, MD, brought to you by the SVS History Project Work Group.

 http://tinyurl.com/CambriaXR

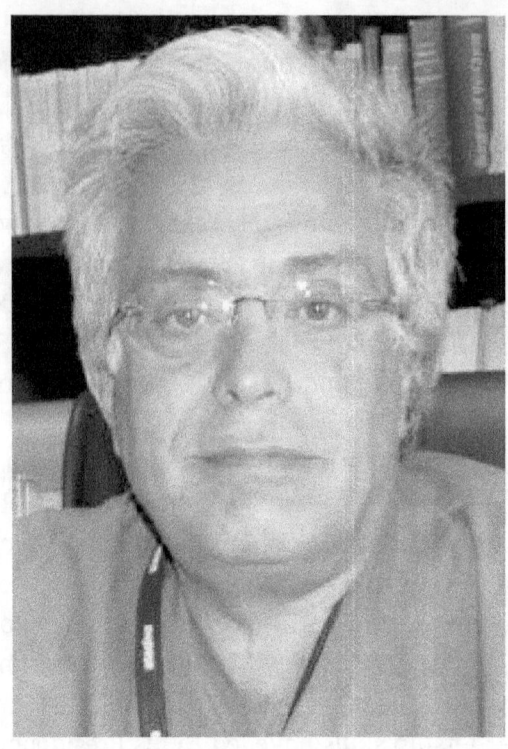

Piergiorgio Cao, MD

Piergiorgio Cao is an Italian vascular surgeon, surgical leader, educator and researcher. He was born in Rome on September 29, 1947, and was raised in the city. His father was a lawyer who worked for the National Telephone Company of Italy and his mother was a housewife. He studied medicine at the University La Sapienza in Rome and graduated from medical school in 1972. His general surgery training and vascular surgery training were at the same university, after which he spent 18 months of clinical fellowship in the United States at the Texas Heart Institute of the Baylor Medical College in Houston. Denton A. Cooley was the director, and he became an important mentor for Dr. Cao.

In 1985 Dr. Cao returned to Italy, where he worked with another important mentor, Dr. Paola Fiorani. He was then recruited to the University of Perugia where he became the Chief of Vascular Surgery as well as full professor and director of the training program in vascular surgery. He later moved to Rome to become the Chief of Vascular Surgery at San Camillo Forlanini Hospital between 2009 and 2015.

Dr. Cao's clinical research interest has included important carotid artery trials. He participated in ECST (the European Carotid Surgery Trial, published in *Lancet* in 1998) and NASCET (the North American Symptomatic Carotid Endarerectomy Trial, reported in *The New England Journal of Medicine* on August 15, 1991). Dr. Cao was the principal investigator and first author for the EVEREST trial, which compared eversion to standard carotid endarterectomy and was published in *The Journal of Vascular Surgery* in 2000. More recently, he has been involved in many important trials to study endovascular treatment of abdominal and thoracic aortic aneurysms. Among these, he was the principal investigator and first author for the CAESAR trial comparing endovascular repair to surveillance in small aortic aneurysms. This study was published in the *European Journal of Vascular and Endovascular Surgery* in 2011.

His interest in endovascular surgery led him to develop the first "hybrid" operating room in Italy. He is also the author of more than 350 papers and book chapters. Dr. Cao was the Senior Editor and then the Editor-in-Chief for the *European Journal of Vascular Surgery* over a period of six years. His academic interest and clinical experience has led him to be invited as a speaker at many international vascular meetings and as a visiting professor at multiple medical schools in Europe and in the United States. Dr. Cao is a member of many Italian and international vascular surgery societies including being a Distinguished Fellow of the Society for Vascular Surgery and also a Fellow of the Royal College of Surgeons.

Scan the QR code below or enter the YouTube link to watch the entire interview with Dr. Piergiorgio Cao conducted by Walter J. McCarthy, MD, brought to you by the SVS History Project Work Group.

 http://tinyurl.com/CaoXP9

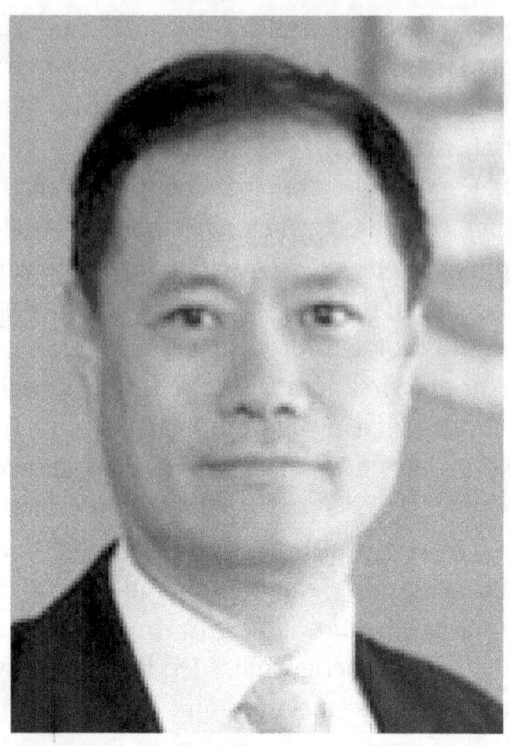

Stephen W.K. Cheng, MD

Professor Stephen Wing-Keung Cheng obtained his qualifications in medicine at the University of Hong Kong in 1984. He received his training in general surgery and vascular surgery from the Queen Mary Hospital Department of Surgery in Hong Kong. In training he was inspired toward a career in vascular surgery by John Wong, who was an early vascular practitioner, and was the Department Chairman there from 1983 until 2008. In 1991, Dr. Cheng was invited to be a visiting Assistant Professor at the University of California, San Francisco, where he went to pursue his special interest in vascular surgery. In San Francisco he trained under Ronald Stoney and Jerry Goldstone, whom he considers mentors. Returning home in 1992, he was appointed Chief of the Division of Vascular Surgery and Director of the Francis Y.H. Tien Vascular Disease Centre and the Vascular Laboratories at the Queen Mary Hospital in Hong Kong. He is currently the Serena H.C. Yang Professor of Vascular Surgery at the University of Hong Kong.

Dr. Cheng's main interest is vascular surgery and endovascular treatment of occlusive and aneurysmal diseases. He is a Distinguished Fellow and Honorary Member of the Society for Vascular Surgery and an Honorary Member of the Australian and New Zealand Society for Vascular Surgery. He is also a member of the European Society for Vascular Surgery, an Executive Board Member and Asian Chapter Secretary of the International Union of Angiology, and a National Representative to the International Society for Vascular Surgery. Dr. Cheng is Past President of the Asian Society for Vascular Surgery and Past Governor of the American College of Surgeons, Hong Kong Chapter.

Dr. Cheng is on the editorial board of the *Chinese Journal of Vascular Surgery* and the *Journal of Vascular Surgery.* He has held Visiting Professorships at the University of British Columbia and at the Imperial College of Science, Technology and Medicine in London.

Professor Cheng played a key role in the development of vascular surgery in Hong Kong, having established a renowned unit and the first non-invasive vascular laboratory at the Queen Mary Hospital. He led the development of endovascular intervention of peripheral vascular disease and endovascular aortic stent grafting for aortic aneurysms and aortic dissection in Southeast Asia. He has been invited to lecture and to lead workshops for advanced endograft techniques in many countries throughout Asia. Professor Cheng's research is also directed toward many aspects of aortic aneurysm and aortic dissection. He has authored more than 200 publications in peer-reviewed journals and book chapters in these and other areas. Dr. Cheng has been the Chairman of the Department of Surgery at Hong Kong University since 2017.

Many of these comments are courtesy of Hong Kong University.

Scan the QR code below or enter the YouTube link to watch the entire interview with Dr. Stephen W.K. Cheng conducted by Peter F. Lawrence, MD, and James S.T. Yao, MD, brought to you by the SVS History Project Work Group.

 http://tinyurl.com/ChengXS1

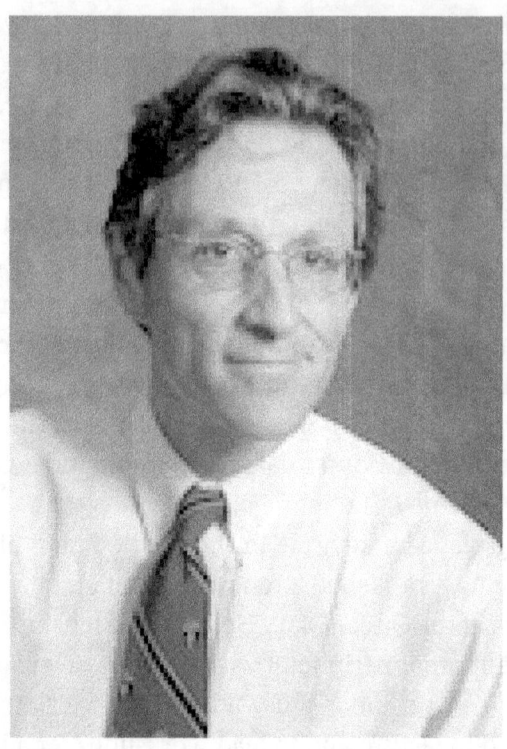

Timothy A.M. Chuter, MD

Timothy Chuter was born in Birmingham, England in 1958. His mother was a nurse and his father a geologist and mining engineer whose work took the family to Africa for many years. The family returned to England in time for Tim to attend high school in Leeds. Dr. Chuter went on to study medicine in Nottingham, graduating in 1982.

He came to America with his wife, who was an actress, and they settled in New York City. Dr. Chuter taught anatomy at Columbia University and became a surgical resident there. After residency, in 1990, he went to Rochester, New York, as a fellow in critical care. This was followed by a fellowship in vascular surgery under Drs. James DeWeese and Richard Green. Afterwards, Dr. Chuter returned to Nottingham to concentrate on research and to begin his MD thesis. He helped start the endovascular program in Nottingham with Dr. Brian Hopkinson.

Dr. Chuter was recruited back to Columbia University, which he considered his surgical home. However, he made many trips to Europe from New York performing endovascular cases with a wide variety of surgeons, and learning many new techniques. These experiences, along with frequent work with interventional radiologists, led Dr. Chuter to develop and refine endovascular graft delivery systems and to design and implant the first bifurcated aortic endovascular grafts. He holds more than 40 patents, 23 related to this work, and he has authored more than 145 journal publications.

Dr. Chuter strongly believes in the importance of collaboration and in the necessity of knowing one's own "gaps," and then recruiting talented people who can fill them. He is very aware of the importance industry plays in getting innovations from inventors to patients. To enhance this process, he has focused on helping industry to be more iterative, refining inventions before rolling out products on a large scale.

Dr. Chuter is currently a Professor of Surgery and Director of the Endovascular Surgery Program at UCSF. Among his many honors, Dr. Chuter was awarded the Society for Vascular Surgery Medal for Innovation in 2008 and the Jacobson Innovation Award from the American College of Surgeons in 2017.

Scan the QR code below or enter the YouTube link to watch the entire interview with Dr. Timothy A.M. Chuter conducted by Roger T. Gregory, MD, and James S.T. Yao, MD, brought to you by the SVS History Project Work Group.

 http://tinyurl.com/ChuterXT

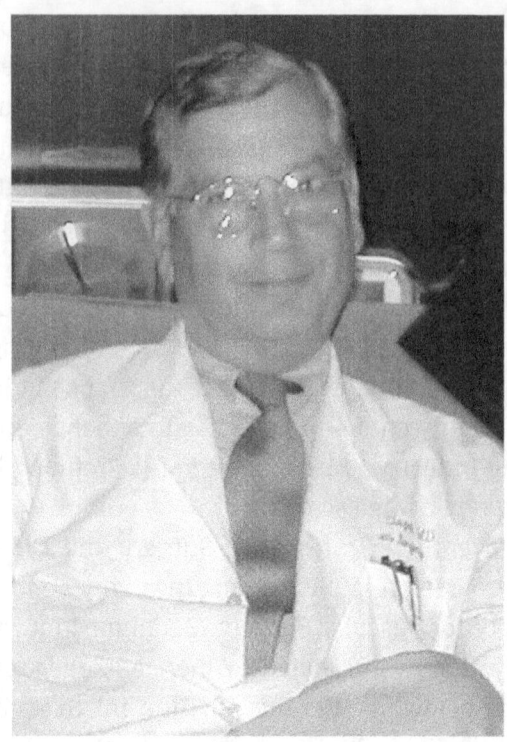

G. Patrick Clagett, MD

G. Patrick Clagett grew up near Washington, DC, in southern Maryland. His father was a lawyer and also a tobacco farmer. He attended a prep school associated with the Annapolis Naval Academy and then selected the University of Virginia for college. He was an English major in college and on graduation was admitted to the University of Virginia for medical school. In the 1960s, after medical school, new physicians were being drafted because of the Vietnam War. However, it was possible to defer service until after completing training through the Berry Plan. Dr. Clagett selected that course and ended up training in general surgery at the University of Michigan. At that time the University of Michigan had a program allowing him to spend two years in Boston conducting animal and clinical research. This exposed him to the issues of venous thromboembolism and platelet biochemistry early in his training.

When he was in surgical training, the University of Michigan Department of Surgery was chaired by William Fry, a pioneer vascular surgeon. In 1976 Dr.

Fry became the Chairman of Surgery at the University of Texas Southwestern in Dallas and eventually recruited Dr. Clagett to his program there. After general surgery, Dr. Clagett selected a Vascular Fellowship in a one-year program at Walter Reed Hospital, where he was mentored by Norman Rich. Following the fellowship, Dr. Clagett was asked to stay on staff at Walter Reed and, due to unexpected circumstances, soon became the Chief of the Vascular Service at a very early stage in his career.

Dr. Clagett eventually moved to Texas Southwestern in 1983 and became the Chief of Vascular Surgery and also Chief at Parkland Hospital. He soon developed a Vascular Fellowship for which he was the Program Director. Between these two institutions he was responsible for all types of vascular surgery. An operation he pioneered and is often remembered for is replacing infected abdominal aortic grafts with femoral vein taken from the patient's thighs. Facing the daunting task of aortic reconstruction after infected abdominal aortic prosthetic graft removal, Dr. Clagett conceived this new technique. He had heard a presentation that discussed using the femoral vein for femoral-popliteal arterial reconstruction and extrapolated the idea to the abdominal aorta. Consulting on a patient with no other possibility of reconstruction, a sentinel patient, he went ahead with this technique and was successful. Using this leap of surgical imagination, he was eventually able to report salvaging numerous patients. This included carefully following their venous complications, which were usually minimal. The new technique was soon adopted around the world providing treatment for many otherwise desperate patients.

During his long career he was responsible for mentoring and training numerous vascular fellows as well as encouraging many general surgery residents from the Texas Southwestern program to go into vascular surgery.

Dr. Clagett has held many important national positions. These include serving as a member of the American Board of Surgery during the difficult time when vascular surgery was attempting to separate from that Board. Dr. Clagett was also elected President of the Society for Vascular Surgery, serving from 2009–2010.

Scan the QR code below or enter the YouTube link to watch the entire interview with Dr. Patrick Clagett conducted by Walter J. McCarthy, MD, brought to you by the SVS History Project Work Group.

 http://tinyurl.com/ClagettXGP

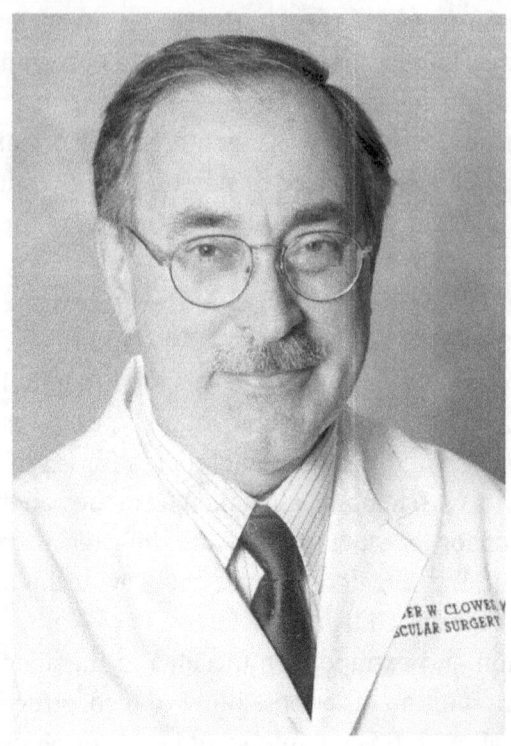

Alexander Whitehill Clowes, MD

Alec Clowes was born in 1946 into a family with a medical and scientific legacy dating back centuries. It can be traced to 1588, when Sir William Clowes, a British Naval surgeon, published one of the earliest textbooks of surgery in the English language. More recently, Alec's grandfather, George Clowes, was Director of the Research Laboratory for the Eli Lilly Company, where he was a driving force behind the mass production of insulin for human use in 1923. Alec's father, George Clowes Jr., was an academic surgeon who practiced at Case Western Reserve and Harvard Medical School. Following the Clowes' tradition, Alec concentrated on science, attending Harvard College (1968) and Harvard Medical School (1972).

Dr. Clowes decided to pursue a career in academic surgery, completing his general surgery training at Case Western Reserve in Cleveland. During residency he was able to take time from training for research and worked in the laboratory of Dr. Morris Karnovsky at Harvard Medical School (1974–1977).

During this time, he developed what would become his lifelong interest in vascular biology. He would soon become fascinated with the then virtually unknown subject of arterial remodeling after injury, particularly "myo-intimal hyperplasia." After surgical residency, he returned to Boston to the Peter Bent Brigham Hospital for vascular surgery training under John Mannick, 1979–1980.

In 1980, Dr. Clowes was recruited to join the faculty of the Department of Surgery at the University of Washington in Seattle. He was attracted to the west coast by the outstanding faculty with expertise in blood vessel-related research at the University of Washington. Dr. Clowes soon rose to Professor of Surgery in 1990, and he was appointed adjunct Professor of Pathology in 1992. From 1992 to 1993 he served as Acting Chairman of the Department of Surgery and was Chief of the Division of Vascular Surgery from 1995 to 2007. He remained at the University of Washington for his entire career.

Throughout his clinical years, Dr. Clowes focused on research and mentoring the younger generation of academic surgeons. He was funded for more than 30 years by the NIH and was a recipient of their MERIT award. As a testament to his leadership and dedication to research, he received the Flance-Karl award given by the American Surgical Association in 2005. He has also received a Lifetime Achievement award from the Society for Vascular Surgery.

Dr. Clowes strongly believed that serious research could be done by vascular surgeons, and he was truly one of the very first fellowship-trained vascular surgeons to achieve this goal. Besides his own clinical and research achievements, some of Dr. Clowes' most significant contributions involved advancing the prospect of research career support for upcoming vascular surgeons. He accomplished this repeatedly by directly establishing or organizing and promoting career development award grants to support basic laboratory research. This funding has been arranged through the American College of Surgeons, the Society for Vascular Surgery and the National Institutes of Health. Dr. Clowes' effort to promote research funding has subsequently been responsible for the careers of numerous vascular surgery researchers and their many important scientific contributions.

Dr. Clowes died of a brain glioblastoma on July 7, 2015, at age 68.

Scan the QR code below or enter the YouTube link to watch the entire interview with Dr. Alexander W. Clowes conducted by Melina R. Kibbe, MD, and William H. Pearce, MD, brought to you by the SVS History Project Work Group.

 http://tinyurl.com/ClowesXA

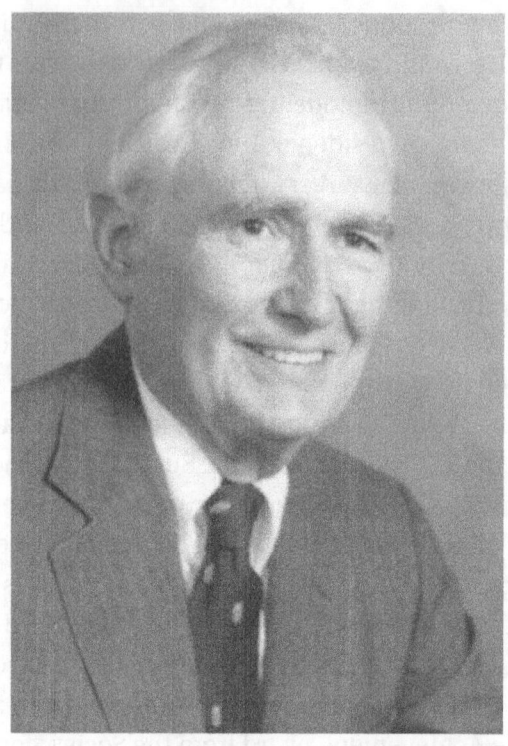

John E. Connolly, MD

John "Jack" Earl Connolly was on born May 21, 1923 in Omaha, Nebraska, where his father practiced surgery and was a faculty member at Creighton University. The children often joined their father on weekend hospital rounds. Jack's brother also went into surgery, becoming a neurosurgeon. Jack attended Harvard College, graduating in 1945, and then went on to Harvard Medical School. During his medical school rotations at the Massachusetts General Hospital, he was fascinated by observing the surgical procedures of Robert Linton and R. Clement Darling Jr., both pioneer vascular surgeons.

After medical school, during his third year of general surgery residency at Stanford, Dr. Connolly decided to be a vascular surgeon. His chairman, Emile Holman, arranged for him to spend a year in London under Sir James Patterson as a Surgical Registrar at St. Bartholomew's Hospital. The young Dr. Connolly was also able to travel in Europe and to meet many of the leading vascular surgeons, who at that time in the early 1950s were inventing arterial reconstructive surgery as we know it today. Dr. Connolly was known later in his career as an important international ambassador of American vascular surgery. He believes this is most likely due to his early travel abroad in England and Europe.

Dr. Connolly subsequently finished general surgery residency at Stanford and went on to two years of thoracic surgery training at Columbia in New York City. He was then recruited back to the Stanford faculty as an Instructor of Surgery in 1957. He was honored by being named a Markle Scholar from 1957 to 1962, during which time he operated and cared for patients, wrote many papers and conducted research on deep hypothermia for brain protection in the dog laboratory. In 1965, Dr. Connolly was recruited to be the Surgical Chairman at the University of California in Irvine. With this appointment he became the founding Department Chairman, completely building the Department, hiring faculty for seven new divisions of surgery and also for anesthesia. He served as Chairman for 13 years and remained clinically active at UC Irvine long afterward.

Dr. Connolly served as President of the International Society of Cardiovascular Surgery, North American Chapter, in 1976. He contributed to the American College of Surgeons as a Governor (1957–1960), a Regent (1972–1983) and in multiple other leadership roles. He is one of the few American surgeons to have been awarded an Honorary Fellowship in the Royal College of Surgeons of England, Edinburgh and Ireland respectively. Former trainees, including those in Japan and South America, established a John E. Connolly Surgical Society in 1975. Among Dr. Connolly's special clinical interests in vascular surgery were the in-situ vein graft and awake carotid surgery. He served as Co-Chair Editor of the journal *Cardiovascular Surgery* for ten years. Dr. Connolly's son, Peter, practices vascular surgery at Cornell University in New York City.

Dr. Jack Connolly died on January 20, 2016 at age 92.

Scan the QR code below or enter the YouTube link to watch the entire interview with Dr. John E. Connolly conducted by Peter F. Lawrence, MD, brought to you by the SVS History Project Work Group.

 http://tinyurl.com/ConnoXJ1

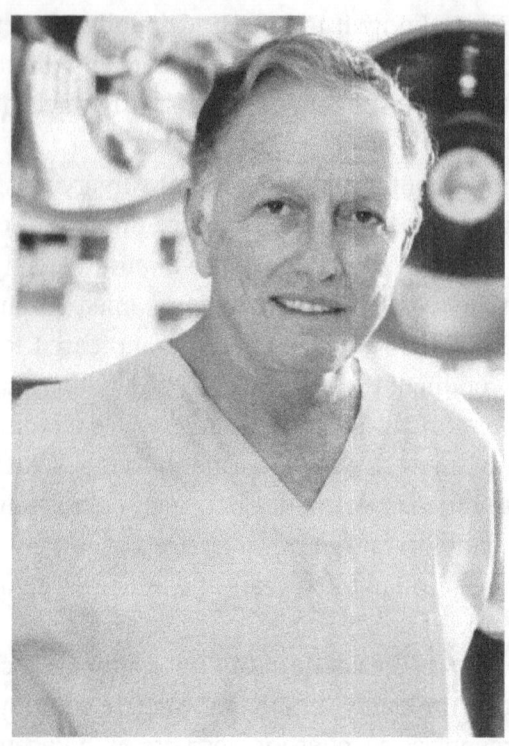

Denton A. Cooley, MD

Denton Cooley was an iconic cardiovascular and vascular surgeon who had trained in these fields at the very beginning of the specialties as we know them today. His surgical training began at Johns Hopkins in 1944 when Alfred Blalock was the chief of surgery there. Dr. Cooley was the intern the day that Dr. Blalock performed the first "blue baby" operation for tetralogy of Fallot.

After general surgery training, Dr. Cooley spent one year in England with Russell Brock, who was then perhaps the most experienced thoracic surgeon in the United Kingdom. Dr. Cooley then was recruited to return to his home town of Houston, Texas in 1951 to join Michael DeBakey in practice at Methodist Hospital. He worked hand-in-hand with Dr. DeBakey for nine years during which fundamental advances in aortic surgery, instrumentation, cardiopulmonary bypass and cardiac valve surgery were made. In 1960 he moved his practice to nearby St. Luke's Episcopal Hospital and soon afterwards founded the Texas Heart Institute in 1962.

It's not possible to briefly encapsulate Dr. Cooley's massive surgical career. Once the Texas Heart Institute was established under his direction, he was able to efficiently operate on many patients every day. It is estimated that he and his team operated on approximately 140,000 patients throughout his career; his personal estimate was that about 20 percent of these were vascular cases. Otherwise, he concentrated on cardiac surgery and also congenital cardiac surgery. His surgical skill, speed and stamina are legendary. He also produced more than 1,400 publications and twelve books related to his experience. Over his long career he mentored and inspired hundreds of surgical trainees. Many of them went on to become world leaders in their specialties.

Dr. Cooley was the first to perform many surgical procedures, including the first long-term successful human-to-human heart transplant in the United States on May 2, 1968. He also placed the first total artificial heart in 1969. The artificial heart had primarily been a project of Michael DeBakey's, and its first-time use by Dr. Cooley led to a disagreement between the two surgeons. They finally resolved their differences in a famous reconciliation in 2007 when Dr. DeBakey was 99 years old.

Dr. Cooley received countless honors throughout his career, among them the René Leriche Prize in 1967 and the Presidential Medal of Freedom from Ronald Reagan in 1984.

In addition to his his surgical speed, skill and calm demenaor in the operating room, Dr. Cooley was also known for his quick wit. He was a life-long golfer and tennis player and played bass in a swing band called "The Heartbeats." He married Louise Thomas in 1949, and together they raised five daughters.

Dr. Cooley died on November 18, 2016, at age 96, at his home in Houston.

Scan the QR code below or enter the YouTube link to watch the entire interview with Dr. Denton A. Cooley conducted by Roger T. Gregory, MD, brought to you by the SVS History Project Work Group.

 http://tinyurl.com/CooleyXD

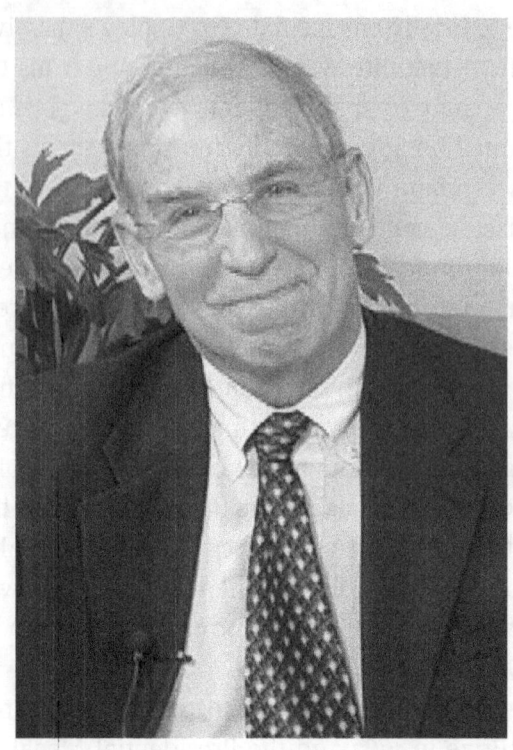

Jack L. Cronenwett, MD

Jack Cronenwett grew up in Ludington, Michigan, a harbor town on the eastern shore of Lake Michigan. His father was a machinist, and together they enjoyed fishing and hunting. In high school Jack always intended to become an electrical engineer and he only applied to engineering schools for college. He ended up at the University of Michigan, but along the way switched majors and graduated as a psychology major. A neurologist with whom he had done summer research successfully convinced him to apply to medical school. He received his MD from Stanford University, having decided on a surgical career. Dr. Cronenwett's general surgery residency was back at the University of Michigan after which he decided to broaden his surgical horizons. Therefore, he entered the vascular fellowship at the University of Tennessee under Dr. Ed Garrett. After fellowship training, he returned to the University of Michigan as a faculty member, but he was soon recruited by Dartmouth Medical School to be their new chief of vascular surgery.

At his new job, besides his surgical responsibilities, Dr. Cronenwett also began work with the Dartmouth Institute for Health Policy and Clinical Practice on outcome analysis and quality improvement in healthcare. His work in this area culminated in a unique book, *The Dartmouth Atlas of Vascular Health Care*. This text, co-authored with John Birkmeyer in 2000, addressed many important issues including the varying rates of vascular healthcare and surgery delivered in different regions of the United States.

During his career, Dr. Cronenwett has served vascular surgery in many senior positions: as member of the Resident Review Committee for Surgery of the ACGME, as President of the New England Society for Vascular Surgery, and as Co-Editor, with James M. Seeger, of the *Journal of Vascular Surgery*. He was also Co-Editor, with K. Wayne Johnston, of *Rutherford's Vascular Surgery* textbook (7th and 8th editions). One of his most significant and most appreciated contributions was a leadership role he played while serving as President of the SVS in 2003 and 2004. At that time, he guided the merger of the SVS and the AAVS (formerly ISCVS-NA) into a single vascular society. Dr. Cronenwett worked in concert with Dr. Tom Riles, who was President of the AAVS during those years, to shepherd the process. The SVS became a single society representing all of the vascular surgeons in North America.

Dr. Cronenwett's organizational skills, combined with his interest in the principles of outcome research led him to develop and oversee the Vascular Study Group of New England, a regional co-operative quality improvement project involving 27 hospitals. Success with this initial regional effort gradually led to an expansion of this concept across all of North America. His program, now called the VQI, the Vascular Quality Initiative, has become immensely important to vascular surgery. The VQI has become fully endorsed and sponsored by the Society for Vascular Surgery, has more than 968 participating surgical centers and recently celebrated enrolling its one millionth patient.

Jack has semi-retired, is learning to play golf and, fortunately, will continue to be involved with the VQI.

Scan the QR code below or enter the YouTube link to watch the entire interview with Dr. Jack L. Cronenwett, MD, conducted by William H. Baker, MD, brought to you by the SVS History Project Work Group.

 http://tinyurl.com/CronenXJ

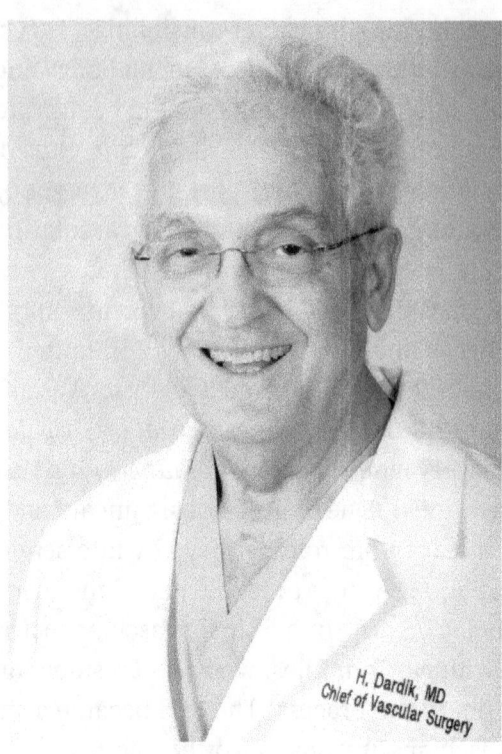

Herbert Dardik, MD

Herbert Dardik was born on May 17, 1935, to Russian immigrants in Long Branch, New Jersey. Dr. Dardik received his medical degree from New York University School of Medicine and completed his surgical residency at Montefiore Medical Center in New York City. He then joined Englewood Hospital in Englewood, New Jersey and eventually served there as Chief of Vascular Surgery and also as Director of the Vascular Fellowship Training Program, which he founded in 1978. During much of his professional life he was a Professor of Surgery at the Mount Sinai School of Medicine.

In addition to always maintaining a busy private clinical practice and teaching, Dr. Dardik sustained a keen interest in academic and research endeavors. His unique idea of using the human umbilical cord as an arterial bypass graft was most innovative. This work won him the Hektoen Gold Medal from the American Medical Association in 1976 and is one of the accomplishments he is often remembered for. Another significant contribution included his idea to sometimes construct an arteriovenous fistula at the distal end of a femoral-distal bypass to improve the graft patency rate. This, thereby, could enhance limb salvage. He also developed an everted cervical vein patch technique for carotid endarterectomy.

Dr. Dardik authored two books, 48 book chapters and 167 articles. He was an invited speaker at many national and international meetings. He served as President of the Society for Clinical Vascular Surgery, the Eastern Vascular Society, and the Vascular Society of New Jersey. In recognition of his many contributions to vascular surgery, the Society for Vascular Surgery granted him its Lifetime Achievement Award in 2017. This was awarded for the first time to a surgeon who truly hailed from private clinical surgical practice rather than from academia.

All three of Dr. Dardik's children are physicians. His son, Alan, is a vascular surgeon at Yale University. Dr. Dardik reflected on the question of when an aging surgeon should stop performing operations while he participated in an in-depth discussion for a *New York Times* article, published on February 1, 2019. He had stopped performing operations of his own volition at age 80, in 2016. Dr. Dardik died on May 11, 2020 at the age of 84.

Scan the QR code below or enter the YouTube link to watch the entire interview with Dr. Herbert Dardik conducted by Melina R. Kibbe, MD, brought to you by the SVS History Project Work Group.

 http://tinyurl.com/DardikXH

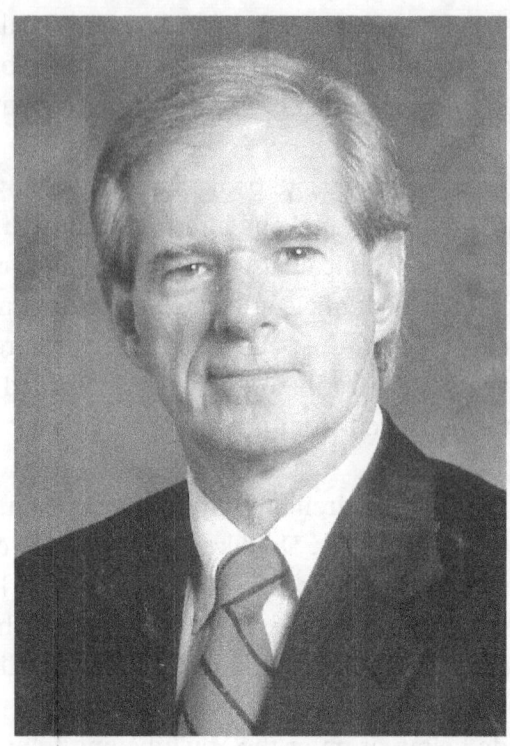

Richard H. Dean, MD

Richard Dean was born in Radford, Virginia in 1942. He received his BA from the Virginia Military Institute and his medical degree from the Medical College of Virginia. After completing a vascular fellowship at Northwestern University, studying under John J. Bergan and James S.T. Yao, he joined the faculty of Vanderbilt University. At Vanderbilt from 1975 until 1986 he rose to Professor and Division Head of Vascular Surgery.

Dr. Dean moved to Wake Forest University (WFU) as Professor and to serve as the Chairman of Surgery in 1987. He was then appointed President and CEO of WFU Health Sciences, Senior VP for Health Affairs of WFU and Director of the WFU Baptist Medical Center from 1997 until retiring in 2007. He is now the President Emeritus of WFU Health Sciences. Dr. Dean has participated on many advisory boards. Notably, while serving on the American Board of Surgery, he was the first to advocate for a "sub-board" structure for vascular surgery, under the umbrella of the American Board of Surgery.

During his busy clinical surgical career, Dr. Dean had expertise in all areas of open vascular surgery, but became best known for his management of renal artery problems. This was at a time when endovascular solutions in this area were not possible. Through the operations that he devised, and subsequently described in publications, he became truly a world leader in the techniques of renal artery bypass, endarterectomy and repair of complex renal artery aneurysms.

During his leadership at Wake Forest University, Dr. Dean spearheaded the development of a 200+ acre urban research park in Winston-Salem. In recognition of his leadership, the Biomedical Research Building was named after him. His many other recognitions include an Honorary Doctorate Degree from the Medical University of Vienna, the Distinguished Alumnus Award from the Medical College of Virginia and the Medallion of Merit from WFU.

Dr. Dean is married to Mary Greene Dean. Between them, they have seven children and ten grandchildren. He enjoys working in his consulting firm, relaxing at his lake house in Virginia and woodworking.

Scan the QR code below or enter the YouTube link to watch the entire interview with Dr. Richard H. Dean, conducted by Mark K. Eskandari, MD, brought to you by the SVS History Project Work Group.

 http://tinyurl.com/DeanXR1

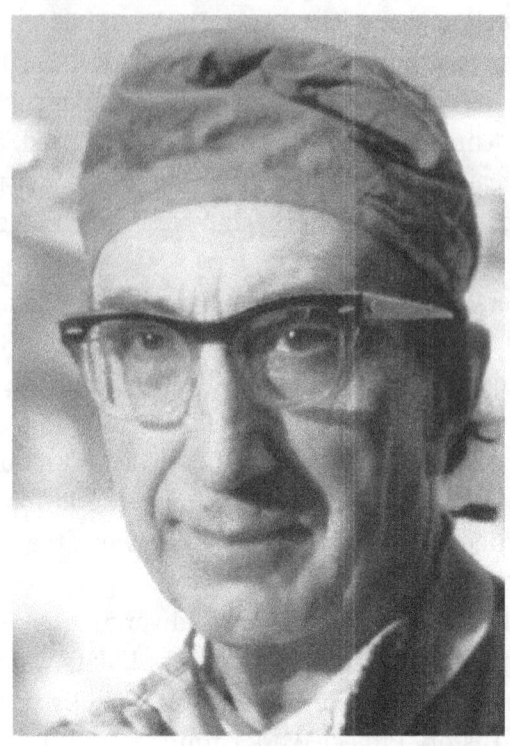

Michael DeBakey, MD

Every vascular surgeon knows of Michael DeBakey (September 7, 1908–July 11, 2008). We use the instruments he invented every day and ask our scrub nurse for them using his name. He lived to be 99 years old and practiced medicine until the end of his life, giving him a career span nearly twice as long as most surgeons. He trained more than 1000 surgeons. Many of us were trained by him, were trained by surgeons he had trained, had met him, or had heard him speak Dr. DeBakey's life was filled with remarkable achievements, not only related to the innovation and the advancement of vascular and cardiac surgery as we know it today, but also in many other areas. For example, as a young man during World War II, he was an important medical consultant and later a historian of vascular surgery during that conflict. During his career he oversaw the development of the Houston Medical Center and led Baylor University in many roles. He was a trusted consultant to presidents of the United States. He operated on foreign heads of state in their home countries. He was a founding member of the Society for Vascular Surgery in 1947 and was later president. He became the first editor-in-chief of the *Journal of Vascular Surgery* in 1984. Dr. DeBakey received every high honor imaginable, has a society and a surgical department named for him, and a museum in Houston related to his career. Of vascular and cardiac surgeons in the 20th century, no one contributed more or has a higher stature than Michael DeBakey.

If one wishes to learn more about Michael DeBakey, either as a fellow surgeon or as a historian, there is much written material. However, it is very important to actually see and listen to him and his colleagues. The video material available through the Society for Vascular Surgery website is a remarkable chance to hear the great man himself discuss his upbringing, career, philosophy, and the events of surgical history. Also of great interest, the video tour of the Michael DeBakey Museum in Houston includes a session with three of his closest surgical associates who discuss his life and work. The seven separate videos can be easily viewed scanning the QR codes below.

F. William Blaisdell, MD, who was trained by Michael DeBakey, interviews him at the time of the 50th anniversary of the Society for Vascular Surgery in 1997.

 http://tinyurl.com/DeBXB50

Roger Gregory, who was also trained by Michael DeBakey, and is a past president of the Michael DeBakey Society, interviews Dr. DeBakey, specifically focusing on his memories of Rudolph Matas.

 http://tinyurl.com/DeBXRM1

Members of the History Project Work Group, including Roger Gregory, Richard Lynn, Walter McCarthy, and James Yao traveled to Houston on October 24–25, 2016, to visit the Michael DeBakey Museum. The museum tour was led by Kenneth Mattox. Later, the Work Group was able to interview Kenneth Mattox, Charles McCollum and George Noon to discuss Dr. DeBakey's life in detail. Subsequently, Jan Muller, the History Project's videographer, returned to Houston to photograph the museum in more detail before preparation of the final video. Scan the QR code below or enter the YouTube link to watch the entire guided tour of the Michael E. DeBakey Library/Museum in Houston, TX, conducted by Roger T. Gregory, MD, James S.T. Yao, MD, William T. Butler, MD, Kenneth L. Mattox, MD, George P. Noon, MD, and Charles H. McCollum, MD.

 https://tinyurl.com/DeBXMuT

Scan the QR code below or enter the YouTube link to watch a scrolling list of all of Dr. Michael E. DeBakey's Honorary Degrees and Honors.

 https://tinyurl.com/DeBXHon

Scan the QR code below or enter the YouTube link to watch the background of how the Michael E. DeBakey Library/Museum in Houston, TX, was developed with JoAnn Pospisil, MA, BA, and Mary Allen.

 https://tinyurl.com/DeBXMuD

Scan the QR code below or enter the YouTube link to watch the background of how the Michael E. DeBakey Library/Museum video project came about with James S.T. Yao, MD, including an explanation of how the history project work group originated.

 https://tinyurl.com/DeBXPrD

Scan the QR code below or enter the YouTube link to watch the entire discussion of the career of Michael E. DeBakey with colleagues Kenneth L. Mattox, MD, George P. Noon, MD, and Charles H. McCollum, MD, interviewed by Roger T. Gregory, MD, Richard A. Lynn, MD, Walter J. McCarthy, MD, and James S.T. Yao, MD, at the Michael E. DeBakey Library/Museum in Houston, TX.

 https://tinyurl.com/DeBXRem

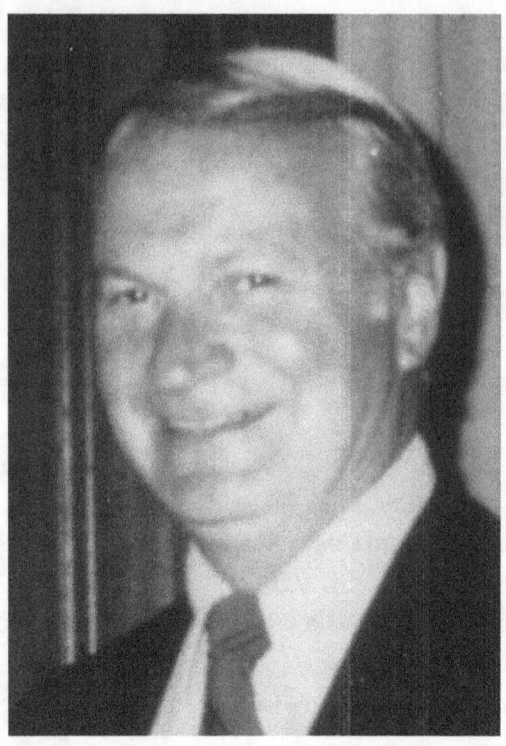

James Arville DeWeese, MD

James A. DeWeese (April 5, 1925–November 14, 2013) was born and raised in Kent, Ohio, and grew up across from Kent State University. His mother was a teacher and his father was a general practice physician who saw patients in the front room of their home. Jim was the youngest of four children. His two older brothers became physicians, and his sister married a surgeon. Jim knew he wanted to be a doctor by the time he graduated from Kent State University High School in 1942. The high school was a small one and nearly everyone participated in sports. He played on the football, basketball and golf teams. Golf ended up becoming a lifelong pursuit and pleasure.

Jim was an excellent student and was accepted with a scholarship to Harvard University. By taking an accelerated course load he accumulated one and one-half year's-worth of credit after his first year in Cambridge. While working at home during summer vacation following his freshman year, Jim was chopping wood and sustained a serious eye injury from a flying wood chip.

He had retinal hemorrhage and retinal detachment and was operated on at the Cleveland Clinic. As part of his recovery, he stayed home the next year. He was able to take additional coursework at Kent State. Jim was disqualified from the military because of the injury; however, with World War II raging, students could be accepted into medical school after having completed only two and one-half years of undergraduate work. Therefore, he began attending Rochester University Medical School, starting in the fall of 1944.

This began a lifelong affiliation with Rochester University. The young doctor DeWeese stayed after medical school to be a surgical resident and then was accepted onto the faculty. His early career spanned the rapid development of vascular surgery and cardiac surgery during the 1950s and 1960s. As a resident, he recalls, he was responsible for procuring aortic tissue from autopsies, cleaning it with antibiotic solution, freeze drying it, and then freezing it to -30°C for later use to repair aortic aneurysms. As a young attending, he recalls using whole-body hypothermia for simple open-heart procedures before pump oxygenators were available. Cooling to 30°C allowed 10–15 minutes of safe cerebral ischemia, which enabled, for example, opening the atrium to suture close an atrial septal defect.

Dr. Charles Rob came from London to be the chief of surgery at the University of Rochester in 1960. Dr. DeWeese worked well with Dr. Rob, and during Dr. Rob's 18-year chairmanship, Dr. DeWeese was made the chief of cardiovascular surgery. Later, he also became the chief of vascular surgery.

During his career, besides maintaining a busy teaching and operative schedule across every type of vascular and cardiac surgery, Dr. DeWeese became a national and internationally known surgical leader. He became the president of many societies, including both the Society for Vascular Surgery and the North American chapter of the International Society for Cardiovascular Surgery. He was also the president of the International Society for Vascular Surgery and the American Venous Forum, among others.

President Lyndon Johnson established a "battle" against cancer, heart disease, and stroke in 1969. As part of this project, Dr. DeWeese was asked to be the chairman of a committee that would look at the optimal resources needed to perform excellent vascular surgery. His committee, including Drs. F. William Blaisdell and John Foster, met with representatives of the American Heart Association and others. The committee concluded that the way to best improve the quality of vascular surgery was to have it performed by surgeons who had been specially trained and certified in that area. It was suggested that certification should be developed by the American Board of Surgery and possibly the American Board of Thoracic Surgery. Dr. DeWeese presented these recommendations to the two vascular societies during the 1972 joint meetings.

During those meetings, which were held in Carmel, California, a resolution was adopted that it was appropriate to have a special certificate for vascular surgery. Dr. DeWeese, who was secretary of the SVS from 1972 until 1976, was responsible for writing a letter to the American Board of Surgery stating the resolution. It wasn't until 1984 that the American Board of Surgery decided to offer a certificate of special competency in general vascular surgery. It was also established in 1984 that the residency review committee (RRC) for surgery could accredit vascular fellowships.

Dr. DeWeese with his colleague, James Adams, is often remembered for developing a device for partial vena cava occlusion to prevent pulmonary embolism. This device—called the Adams-DeWeese vena cava clip—was introduced in 1966. The U-shaped device, made of 2mm thick Teflon plastic with a smooth lower arm and a serrated upper arm, was designed to partially block the vena cava, leaving four small channels to allow blood flow. It could be quite easily placed with a short right flank. The Adams-DeWeese clip had widespread use for approximately 15 years until internal vena cava filter devices of the Greenfield type became available.

Dr. DeWeese's most important contribution to the history of vascular surgery came through editorial work with his friend, George Johnson. They completed a major interview history initiated by Andrew Dale to produce an outstanding text entitled *Band of Brothers, Creators of Modern Vascular Surgery*. The book was copyrighted in 1996 and compiled of edited transcripts of interviews with 37 pioneer vascular surgeons who Dr. Dale had selected and interviewed. Dr. Dale had conducted the tape-recorded interviews in the late 1980s, and when he learned of his own impending death from leukemia, asked George Johnson and Dr. DeWeese to finish up the project. They interviewed a few individuals who were still on the list and completed the editing.

Dr. DeWeese passed away in 2013. He was survived by his wife of many years, Pat. Together they had six children and many grandchildren.

Scan the QR code below or enter the YouTube link to watch the entire interview with Dr. James A. DeWeese conducted by James T. Adams, MD, brought to you by the SVS History Project Work Group.

 http://tinyurl.com/DeWXJ2

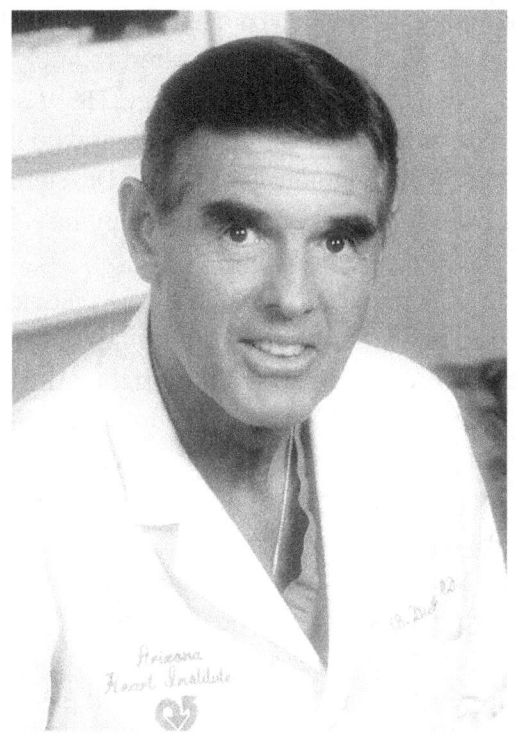

Edward B. Diethrich, MD

Edward B. Diethrich was raised in Hillsdale, a small southern Michigan town, 70 miles from Ann Arbor. He was born on August 6, 1935 at the hospital in Toledo, Ohio where his mother worked as an OR scrub nurse. He was deeply influenced by both of his parents. His father was a coach and a teacher who instilled a love of sports and teamwork. His mother, as a surgical nurse, allowed Ted to observe surgery as a youngster while she cared for patients in the OR at Hillsdale Community Hospital.

Dr. Deithrich attended the University of Michigan in Ann Arbor where he played the trumpet in the marching band. He went on to medical school at Michigan, graduating in 1960. He married his wife Gloria, who he had met in high school, while he was in college.

Dr. Diethrich never considered any specialty other than surgery and completed his residency at St. Joseph's Mercy Hospital in Ann Arbor. Part of the way through his general surgical training he was able to arrange a vascular surgery rotation with Emerick Szilagyi at Henry Ford Hospital in Detroit. The outstanding experience with Dr. Szilagyi led him to apply to Baylor College of Medicine to work under Dr. Michael DeBakey. He was accepted into the program as the first cardiovascular-thoracic resident who had not come from within the Baylor surgical program. Eventually, Dr. DeBakey gained confidence in his young trainee and asked him to stay on the staff at Baylor where Dr. Diethrich worked from 1967 until 1971.

In 1971, Dr. Deithrich struck off on his own path, moving to Phoenix, Arizona. What he had in mind was starting a program that centered on public education about heart disease. He started the Arizona Heart Institute and the Arizona Heart Foundation, which included an outpatient heart clinic. He also established the world's first diagnostic outpatient catheter lab in 1979. He performed the first heart transplant in Phoenix in 1984 followed by the first heart-lung transplant in Arizona in 1985.

Dr. Deithrich was a major, early advocate for endovascular surgery. In 2000, he performed the first endovascular aortic repair for a ruptured aneurysm. At that time, he generously invited surgeons from across the country and from around the world to the Arizona Heart Institute and personally taught them the nuances of endovascular surgery when it was a very new field. He founded the International Society for Endovascular Therapy and the *Journal of Endovascular Therapy* to advance the field.

Dr. Deithrich was a driven problem-solver when he sensed an unmet need. His early innovation, the Sarns sternal saw, adapted from a Sears and Roebuck saber saw when he was still in Ann Arbor, remains in worldwide use. Dr. Diethrich also formed an ultrasound company and two companies that produced aortic endograft devices.

Dr. Diethrich died of a brain oligodendroglioma on February 23, 2017 at age 81. He believed chronic exposure to radiation in the OR was the cause of his disease.

Scan the QR code below or enter the YouTube link to watch the entire interview with Dr. Edward B. Diethrich, conducted by Roger T. Gregory, MD, James S.T. Yao, MD, and Kenneth J. Cherry, MD, brought to you by the SVS History Project Work Group.

 http://tinyurl.com/DiethXE

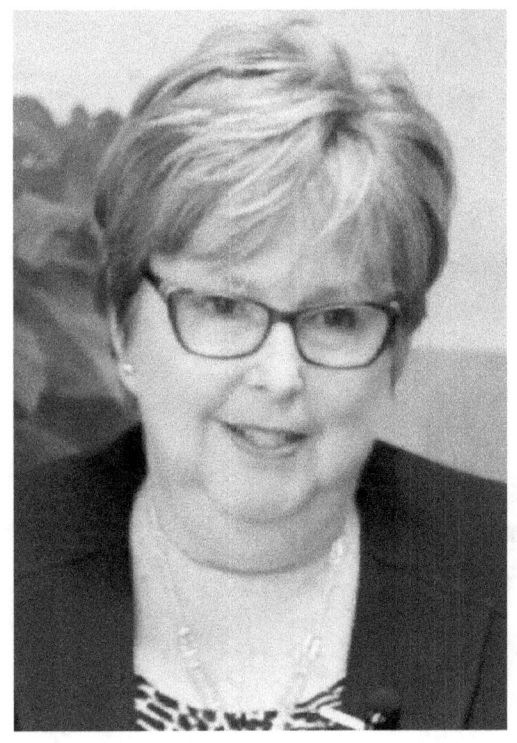 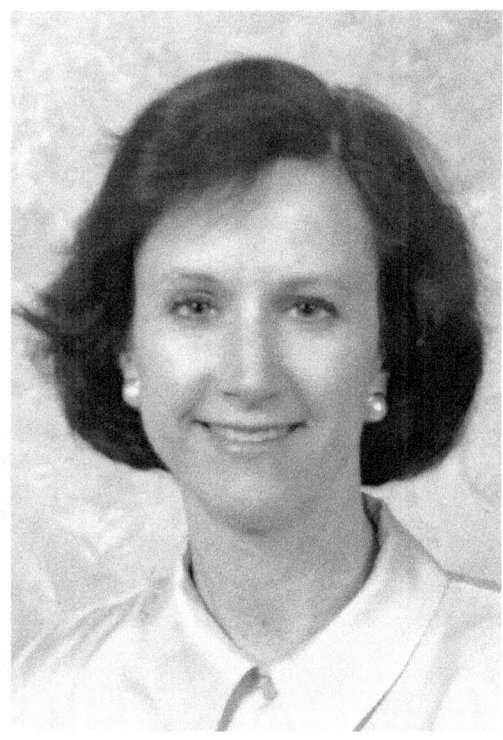

Jeanne Doyle, RN   **Victoria Fahey, RN**

Two of the founding members of the Society for Vascular Nursing discuss the foundations of their society. Starting with eight charter members, and with Jeanne Doyle as the inaugural president, the group held its first regular meeting in 1983 with the Society for Vascular Surgery. The beginnings of the *Journal of Vascular Nursing* and also the first comprehensive vascular nursing textbook, edited by Vicki Fahey, are also explored in this interview.

 http://tinyurl.com/SVNX1

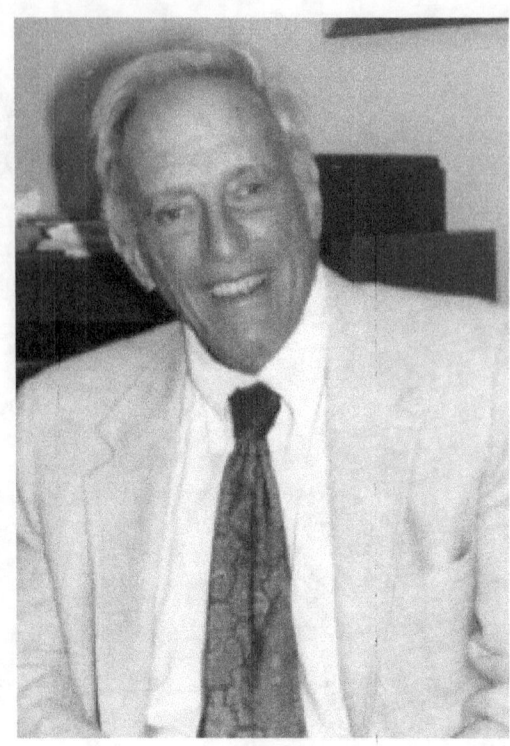

Ben Eiseman, MD

Ben Eiseman was born in St. Louis, Missouri on November 2, 1917. He attended Yale University, graduating in 1939. He went on to Harvard Medical School, finishing in 1943, and into an internship at Massachusetts General Hospital. Immediately afterward, with World War II raging, he joined the U.S. Navy Medical Corps Amphibious Corps. He participated in five invasions as a beach battalion doctor and surgeon, including the Battle of Normandy in June, 1944. His unit then participated in invasions in the Mediterranean and the Pacific theaters. He also served on active duty in Korea, Vietnam and the Gulf War. He retired in 1974 as a Rear Admiral in the Naval Reserve. To honor his service, the surgical ICU at the Veterans Affairs Medical Center at the University of Colorado, where he was Professor Emeritus of Surgery and Medicine, was named after him in September, 1993.

After World War II, Dr. Eiseman was accepted for surgical residency at Barnes Hospital at the Washington University School of Medicine in St. Louis under Dr. Evarts Graham from 1946–50. From there he went on to be Chief of Surgery at the Denver Veterans Administration Hospital (1953–61), then became the founding Chairman of Surgery at the University of Kentucky (1961–67), and eventually returned to Denver to be the founding Chief of Surgery at Denver General Hospital (1967–77). Among his other leadership roles, he served as president of the Society of University Surgeons in 1962. Dr. Eiseman was also Vice President of the American Surgical Association (1982–84) and of the American College of Surgeons (1985–86).

Most notably, Dr. Eiseman was an inspiration, a teacher and a mentor to generations of surgeons. He also conducted research across a truly remarkable spectrum of topics. His more than 450 published articles appeared in a host of surgical and medical journals. A remarkable chapter of his research involved the development of Gore-Tex vascular grafts, as we now know them. This began with an encounter with his good friend Bill Gore, founder of WL Gore. The Eisemans and the Gores had rented a cabin together for skiing at Vail in 1970. Over drinks after a day of skiing, Bill Gore showed Dr. Eiseman a gray neck tie which was made of a new fabric composed of expanded Teflon called Gore-Tex. First, he put mustard on the tie and then demonstrated how easily it could be wiped off. Next, Mr. Gore lit a match and blew a puff of air through the fabric, putting out the match. He then poured water on the tie, showing that the water did not seep through the material. Dr. Eiseman was impressed. He had been working on potential prosthetics for venous and arterial conduits, and he asked if Mr. Gore could make the material into tubes. After experimentation with the material related to fabric pore size and fabric thickness based on trials in dogs and pigs, workable grafts were prepared. The first worldwide human case was soon performed in Denver: Dr. Eiseman implanted a 9mm tube of the new material to allow resection of a portal vein infiltrated with pancreatic cancer. The case was successful, and the patient lived for four years, eventually dying of heart disease.

Dr. Eiseman was awarded the distinction of Honorary Fellow of the Royal College of Surgery (England) in 1990, the Royal College of Surgeons in Thailand and the Columbian College of Surgeons.

In addition, Dr. Eiseman was an accomplished mountaineer who had summited many mountains worldwide including all of the 54 peaks in Colorado with elevations above 14,000 feet. He also participated in Himalayan and Tibetan Plateau Medical Support Expeditions to the East Face of Mount Everest in 1983, Mustagh Ata in 1985, and to K-2 in 1986.

Dr. Eiseman was also once Chairman of the Board of Colorado Outward Bound and Founder of the Tenth Mountain Trail Association.

Dr. Eiseman married Mary Harding in 1945. They had met in England just before D-Day. Together they raised four children. Dr. Eiseman died on November 19, 2012, at age 95.

Scan the QR code below or enter the YouTube link to watch the entire interview with Dr. Ben Eiseman conducted by Norman M. Rich, MD, William H. Pearce, MD, and W. Gerald Rainer, MD, brought to you by the SVS History Project Work Group.

 http://tinyurl.com/EisemanXB

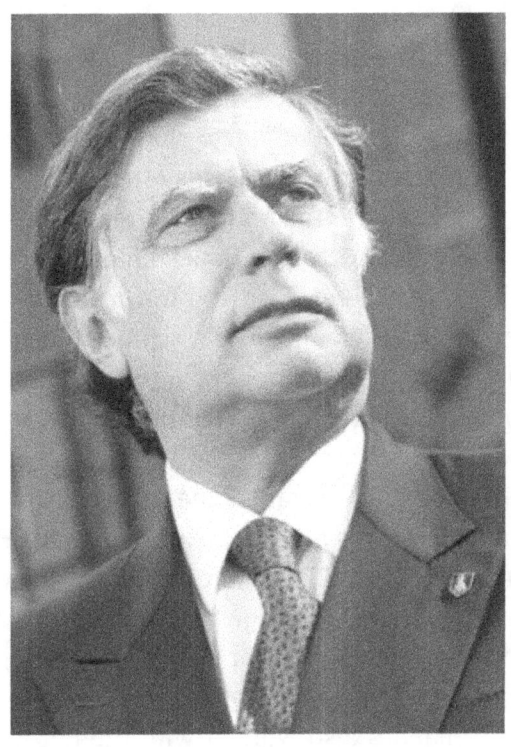

José Fernandes e Fernandes, MD

José Fernandes e Fernandes was raised in a medical family and passed on the tradition of studying medicine to his children. José was born in Portugal. His father was a general practitioner, and his uncle was a surgeon. His mother was a teacher of English and German and endowed him with a lifelong love of reading and literature. His wife was a hospital doctor who put aside her career to raise their two children, both of whom also became physicians. His son, a vascular surgeon, married an ophthalmologist, and his daughter, a pediatrician, married outside of medicine to an engineer of robotics.

Dr. Fernandes e Fernandes knew as early as age nine that he wanted to be a doctor, after observing his uncle perform an appendectomy. Many years later, his uncle developed an aortic aneurysm, and Dr. Fernandes e Fernandes repaired it endovascularly when his uncle was 94 years old.

Dr. Fernandes e Fernandes' surgical training was at the University of Lisbon. He was a resident of the pioneering surgeon Dr. João Cid dos Santos, who had introduced venous phlebography in 1936 and performed the first arterial endarterectomy in 1946, and he was the chairman of surgery at Lisbon University. Dr. dos Santos wrote a letter recommending Dr. Fernandes e Fernandes to travel to St. Mary's Hospital in London to work with the renowned surgeon Felix Eastcott. He recalls that Professor Eastcott taught him the "art and craft" of vascular surgery while he was in London. He spent three years there doing clinical work and research in the blood flow laboratory from 1972–75. During that time, he and his wife were married and his first child was born.

Dr. Fernandes e Fernandes credits his early time at Lisbon University Hospital with preparing him for the endovascular era. In the 1970s he had performed angiography, phlebography and lymphography, which gave him excellent catheter experience.

Dr. Fernandes e Fernandes remembers the early days of endovascular surgery in Portugal in the 1990s as a time of slow adoption. He led the way by performing the first EVAR and TEVAR in the country. He was very involved in promoting vascular science in Europe via the European Society for Vascular Surgery, where he served as President in 1996–97, hosting the annual meeting in Lisbon in 1997.

Dr. Fernandes e Fernandes also worked with the European Union of Specialist Doctors in Brussels, setting training and certification guidelines, and developing a uniform European exam. In his role as Chairman of the Department of Surgery and Dean of the Medical School at the University of Lisbon, Dr. Fernandes e Fernandes pushed for reform in medical studies. He engaged an international committee to recommend reforms that were implemented, including the addition of new medical specialties.

Scan the QR code below or enter the YouTube link to watch the entire interview with Dr. José Fernandes e Fernandes, conducted by Kenneth J. Cherry, MD, and James S.T. Yao, MD, brought to you by the SVS History Project Work Group.

 http://tinyurl.com/FernanXJ

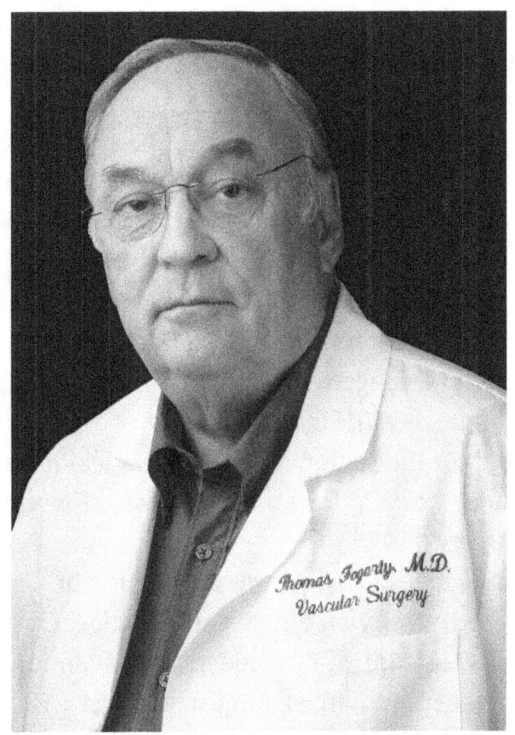

Thomas J. Fogarty, MD

Thomas J. Fogarty began innovating and problem solving at an early age. His development of the Fogarty embolectomy catheter came about during medical school while he was working as an assistant to the pioneer vascular surgeon, Dr. Jack Cranley. Dr. Cranley became a lifelong mentor and was the one who had originally encouraged Dr. Fogarty to consider medical training.

Born in Cincinnati on February 25, 1934, Dr. Fogarty discovered in himself an interest and talent for innovation early in life, repairing things around his mother's home, working on soapbox derby cars, and even building a model-airplane flying wing. As a teenager, he conceived his first major invention, a centrifugal clutch for small gasoline engines which is still in worldwide use today. Tom's father died when he was seven, and with his mother supporting three children by working at a dry cleaners, money was "tight." Young Tom, whose nickname was "Spider" because of his looks, developed a keen interest in boxing. He participated in the Golden Gloves boxing program and also had some professional fights. Among his many jobs to make money for the family, he began working at age 14 cleaning surgical instruments at Good Samaritan Hospital in Cincinnati.

A few years later, while working as a scrub tech at the hospital, he met Dr. Cranley. With Dr. Cranley's friendship and encouragement he gave up boxing and ended up attending Xavier University in Ohio, earning a BS in biology in 1956. This was followed by medical school at the University of Cincinnati College of Medicine. He went on to the University of Oregon where he did his internship and surgical residency from 1962–65. His surgical chairman was J. Englebert Dunphy, who arranged additional training for him. Dr. Fogarty took a two-year fellowship at the NIH in cardiac surgery during his residency. After returning to Portland for the senior year of his surgical residency, he accepted a position on the faculty of Stanford University where Norman Shumway was the Professor of Surgery.

There followed a career of busy surgical practice in vascular and cardiac surgery both at the University and in private practice. Overlying his practice was a nearly nonstop stream of new ideas and inventions, many of which have become important commercial surgical products. His creative, independent spirit, which allowed him to create many medical devices, also led to him founding the Fogarty Institute for Innovation in Mountain View, California in 2007. The Institute's mission is to enable both physicians and engineers to imagine and then develop medical devices and techniques, and finally to commercialize them for use in the market. Dr. Fogarty himself holds over 160 patents.

For his numerous contributions he has been bestowed many honors. These include being named President of the Society for Vascular Surgery in 1995–1996. In 2014, Dr. Fogarty received the National Medal of Technology and Innovation from President Obama at the White House.

Dr. Fogarty founded the Fogarty Winery in 1978 in the Portola Valley in the Santa Cruz Mountains of Northern California. He and his wife raised a daughter and three sons who have gone on to excel in a wide variety of fields.

Scan the QR code below or enter the YouTube link to watch the entire interview with Dr. Thomas J. Fogarty conducted by Melina R. Kibbe, MD, Roger Gregory, MD, and James S.T. Yao, MD, brought to you by the SVS History Project Work Group.

 http://tinyurl.com/FogartyXT

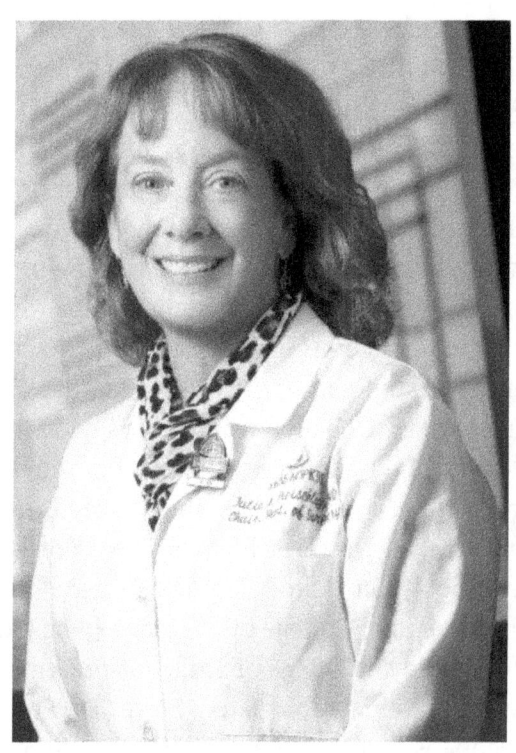

Julie Ann Freischlag, MD

Julie Ann Freischlag was born in 1955 in Decatur, Illinois, the daughter of a teacher mother and newspaper businessman father. At age six, her grandfather told her she could accomplish anything and everything. This has proved to be providential. College at the University of Illinois led to medical school at Rush Medical College in Chicago. Trained in general surgery and vascular surgery at UCLA under Wesley Moore, Dr. Freischlag's first academic positions were in California.

She was recruited back to the Midwest to the Medical College of Wisconsin by Jonathan Towne. This early career foundation led her to return to Los Angeles to become the Chief of Vascular Surgery at UCLA and then eventually to Baltimore to become the Chairman of Surgery at Johns Hopkins University. There she was the first woman to be Chair and was the William Stewart Halsted Professor of Surgery. Later she moved to California to become the Dean of the Medical School at University of California, Davis. Most recently, she has been recruited to be the CEO of the Wake Forest Baptist Health Center in Winston-Salem, North Carolina, where she also serves as the Dean of the Wake Forest School of Medicine.

Everywhere she has been, Dr. Freischlag has advocated for cultural change, including a general sense of fairness, the creation of more opportunities for up-and-coming surgeons and a focus on the importance of outcome research. Dr. Freischlag is known for her frankness in discussing methods of overcoming obstacles and is very open in acknowledging all the mentors and collaborators who have taught her lessons as a clinician and an administrator.

Throughout her leadership career, Dr. Freischlag has always remained a practicing vascular surgeon. One area where she is widely known as a world expert and is the editor of a definitive textbook is in the diagnosis and treatment of the thoracic outlet syndrome. Among many other leadership positions and accomplishments, Dr. Freischlag has been President of the Society for Vascular Surgery (2013), the editor of JAMA Surgery (2005–2014) and was the President of the American College of Surgeons (2021–2022). She has also been inducted into The Royal College of Surgeons of Edinburgh.

This distinguished and remarkable career leaves Dr. Freischlag, a true clinical operating surgeon, as a uniquely experienced leader related to academic medicine, medical education and medical business. In many of her most important accomplishments, she was the very first woman to ever achieve them. Her career, demeanor and philosophy are an inspiration to surgeons, women and men alike. Dr. Freischlag is married to Phil Roethle, a financial executive.

Scan the QR code below or enter the YouTube link to watch the entire interview with Dr. Julie Ann Freischlag conducted by Walter J. McCarthy, MD, and Melina R. Kibbe, MD, with an introduction by James S.T. Yao, MD, brought to you by the SVS History Project Work Group.

 http://tinyurl.com/FreisXJA

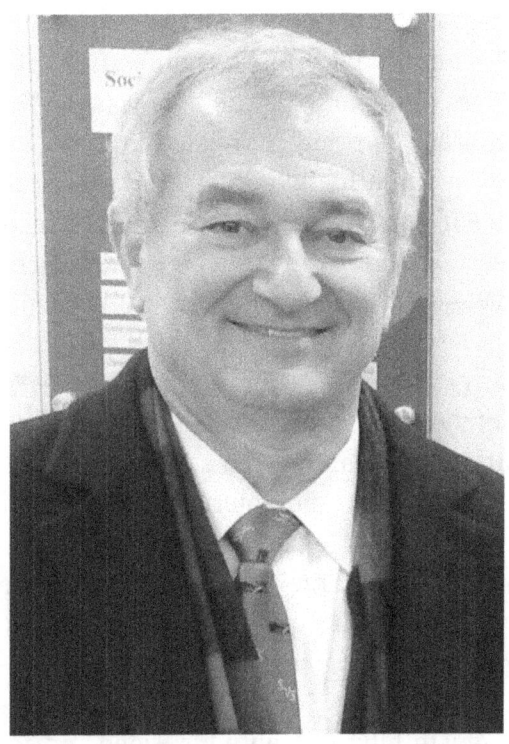

Peter Gloviczki, MD

Peter Gloviczki has spent most of his professional career at the Mayo Clinic in Rochester, Minnesota. He was born in 1948 and raised in northeast Hungary, where his father was a board-certified internist and neurologist. Many other family members were physicians, and a family friend, a surgeon, influenced young Peter toward that specialty. At the age of six he was asked what he wanted to be, and he said he wanted to be a professor of surgery!

Despite being raised in a communist country, Dr. Gloviczki was able to obtain a fine education through the Benedictine High School of the Abbey of Pannonhalma. His excellent grades there led him to a six-year program at Semmelweis University in Budapest where he finished with his medical degree.

During his surgical residency, he was mentored by the pioneer Hungarian vascular surgeon, Professor Lajos Soltesz. Professor Soltesz established the first Hungarian board examination for vascular surgery separate from general surgery in 1980. Additional surgical training in Paris eventually led Dr. Gloviczki to the Mayo Clinic in 1981 where he was the first research fellow under Dr. Larry Hollier. His research, related to major vein and lymphatic reconstruction, resulted in a lifetime interest in those topics. His desire to remain and practice in the United States required a second surgical training in general surgery, so that by the time he began practice in Rochester in 1987, he had completed two full general surgical residencies and three vascular fellowships!

This extensive surgical training led to a practice at the Mayo Clinic across the full spectrum of vascular surgery. This included all areas of arterial, venous and lymphatic surgery, and also a special interest in abdominal and thoraco-abdominal aneurysms, mesenteric and reno-vascular surgery, critical limb ischemia and included bypasses using a microscope. He is an expert on surgical reconstruction of large veins, vascular malformations, chronic venous insufficiency and chylous and lymphatic disorders.

Dr. Gloviczki eventually became the Division Chair of Vascular Surgery at the Mayo Clinic (2000–2010). He became the Editor-in-Chief of the *Journal of Vascular Surgery* in July, 2016 with his friend and colleague Peter Lawrence. Dr. Gloviczki has been the president of many important vascular societies including the Society for Vascular Surgery (2012–2013) and the American Venous Forum (2002–2003). He also has been awarded many international and national awards for his leadership and expertise, including being named the first Edwin Jack Wiley traveling fellow of the Society for Vascular Surgery. He has been made an honorary member of 20 national and international surgical societies and was awarded the Medal of the City of Paris by the mayor in 2006.

The University of Washington in Seattle established the Peter Gloviczki Professorship in Venous and Lymphatic Disorders. His alma mater awarded him the "Doctor Honoris Causa" degree and the "Semmelweis Budapest Award," and he received the Officer's Cross of the Order of Merit of the Republic of Hungary.

Dr. Gloviczki has mentored more than 85 categorical vascular surgery fellows and 25 research fellows. He has edited many vascular textbooks including multiple editions of the outstanding and definitive *Handbook of Venous and Lymphatic Disorders*. He was the associate editor of *Rutherford's Vascular Surgery* for five editions of that classic text. In addition, he himself has authored more than 450 peer-reviewed publications and 250 book chapters.

Dr. Gloviczki is also a highly skilled magician. When he was a ten-year-old, he met a magician who became his mentor, and he soon become a national phenomenon in Hungary: he was known on television as the "small magician." Dr. Gloviczki will occasionally demonstrate his remarkable skills in this area at surgical meetings!

Scan the QR code below or enter the YouTube link to watch the entire interview with Dr. Peter Gloviczki conducted by Mark K. Eskandari, MD, brought to you by the SVS History Project Work Group.

 http://tinyurl.com/GlovXP

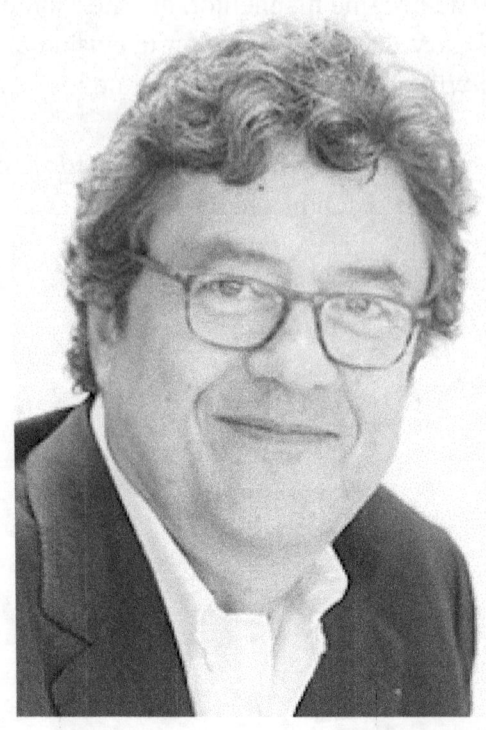

Olivier Goëau-Brissonnière, MD, PhD

Olivier Goëau-Brissonnière was born in Paris on January 6, 1952. He received his MD in Paris in 1981 followed by certification in general surgery in 1983 and vascular surgery in 1986. During training he also spent two years in Quebec City, Canada studying graft infections before returning to France.

Dr. Goëau-Brissonnière earned a PhD in biomedical engineering in Compiègne, France in 1987 and by 1990 he had become a Professor of Vascular Surgery at René Descartes University in Paris. In 1996, Dr. Goëau-Brissonnière became Chairman of the Program of Training in Vascular Surgery at the Paris Faculty of Medicine. He later became the head of the Division of Vascular Surgery at the Hôpital Ambroise Paré in Boulogne Billancourt, France.

Dr. Goëau-Brissonnière has long been involved with *The Annals of Vascular Surgery* through his friend and colleague, Edouard Kieffer. He had worked closely with Kieffer, one of the true pioneer French vascular surgeons, for many years and considers him a mentor. Kieffer and Ramon Berguer were the original co-editors of *The Annals.* Now as a co-editor, he also translates articles from English to French, and from French to English for the journal. *The Annals* has not only French and English, but also Spanish and Chinese translations.

Besides his other accomplishments, Dr. Goeau-Brissonniere has served as President of the French Society for Vascular Surgery and also the Fédération des Spécialités Médicales, which is the umbrella organization for all 42 medical specialties in France.

Scan the QR code below or enter the YouTube link to watch the entire interview with Dr. Olivier Goëau-Brissonnière conducted by Roger T. Gregory, MD, and James S.T. Yao, MD, brought to you by the SVS History Project Work Group.

 http://tinyurl.com/GoBriXO1

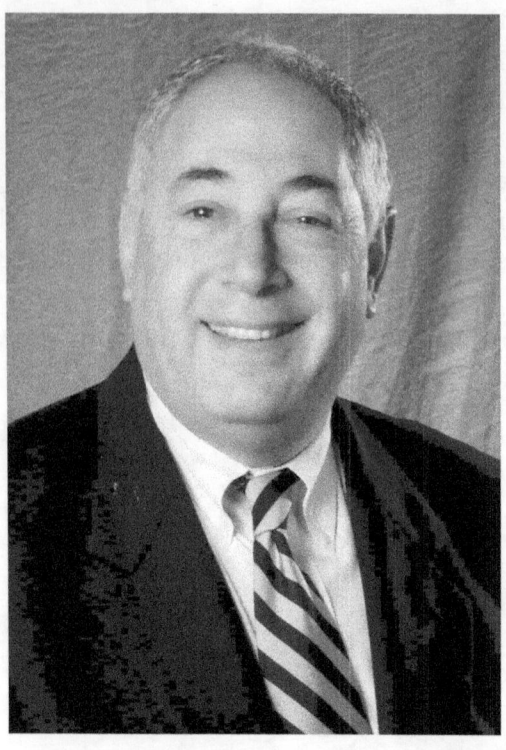

Jerry Goldstone, MD

Jerry Goldstone is an American vascular surgeon who was born on November 18, 1940 in Ontario, Oregon. He attended college at the University of Washington and medical school at the University of Oregon. All of his surgical training was completed at the University of California in San Francisco.

During training, he spent 1968 through 1970 at the Peter Bent Brigham Hospital involved with research related to microcirculation and blood rheology. These topics became a lifelong interest.

As a young attending surgeon, he worked at the University of California, San Francisco VA Hospital for eight years under the direction of Dr. Wesley Moore until 1980. He then accepted a position at the University of Arizona Medical Center in Tucson as the Chief for the Section of Vascular Surgery from 1980 to 1984. He thereafter moved back to the University of California, San Francisco, where he was the Chief of the Division of Vascular Surgery from 1987 to 1995. Moving to the Midwest, he then served as Chief of Vascular

Surgery at the University Hospitals of Cleveland Medical Center until 2008 and became professor emeritus at Case Western Reserve University School of Medicine in 2014. He is currently an adjunct lecturer in the Division of Vascular Surgery at Stanford University.

Dr. Goldstone's many honors include serving as president of many vascular societies including the American Association for Vascular Surgery. He also was named as an Honorary Fellow of the Royal College of Surgeons, Edinburgh. He has co-authored four vascular surgery textbooks and published more than 265 journal articles and book chapters. He is particularly proud of the 51 clinical and research vascular fellows he has taught and mentored during his career.

Scan the QR code below or enter the YouTube link to watch the entire interview with Dr. Jerry Goldstone conducted by Kenneth J. Cherry, MD, and James S.T. Yao, MD, brought to you by the SVS History Project Work Group.

 http://tinyurl.com/GoldstoneXJ

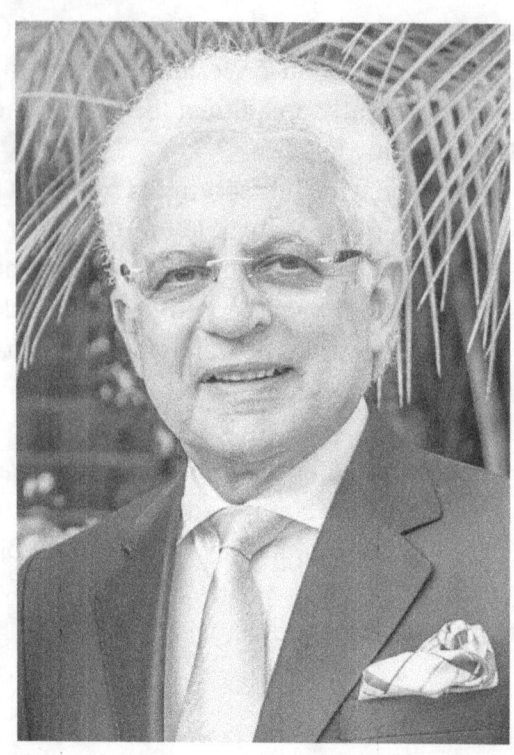

Richard M. Green, MD

Richard Green, a third-generation resident of Rochester, New York, planned to be a doctor even at a young age. After graduation from Colgate University, Green returned to Rochester University School of Medicine and received an MD degree in 1970. He remained there for surgical residency training at Strong Memorial Hospital in Rochester. He was most impressed with Dr. Earle Mahoney, who was chairman of the Department of Surgery and was always hailed as the best surgeon in town. During this period, there were other famous surgeons such as James DeWeese, James May, Andrew Dale, Seymour Schwartz and Charles Rob in the department. Rob, originally from England, was eventually promoted to the surgical chairmanship. Rochester became a powerhouse for general and vascular surgery training.

Dr. Green joined the faculty of Rochester University and with James DeWeese and Charles Rob as mentors, he ascended the academic ladder steadily and eventually became Chairman of Vascular Surgery with full professorship. In 1998, he served as secretary of the SVS and was elected president of the SVS two years later.

One of Dr. Green's major accomplishments as SVS president was his deft handling of negotiations with the American Board of Surgery (ABS). He successfully convinced the ABS to agree to the redefinition of the Vascular Board, removing the need to first have certification in general surgery. As a result, vascular surgery training could be shortened to five years including endovascular technology, non-invasive testing, ultrasound in the vascular laboratory, and imaging techniques such as CT scan and MRI. Consistent with the rule change, the training and practice of vascular surgery was changing dramatically with endovascular technology emerging as a co-dominant modality with open surgery.

In 2013, Dr. Green moved to New York City and became the Chief of the Division of Vascular Surgery at Columbia University. This included being the Associate Chief of the Department of Cardiac, Thoracic and Vascular Surgery. In 2019, he became Professor of Surgery Emeritus at Columbia University.

Scan the QR code below or enter the YouTube link to watch the entire interview with Dr. Richard M. Green conducted by Norman M. Rich, MD, brought to you by the SVS History Project Work Group.

 http://tinyurl.com/GreenXR

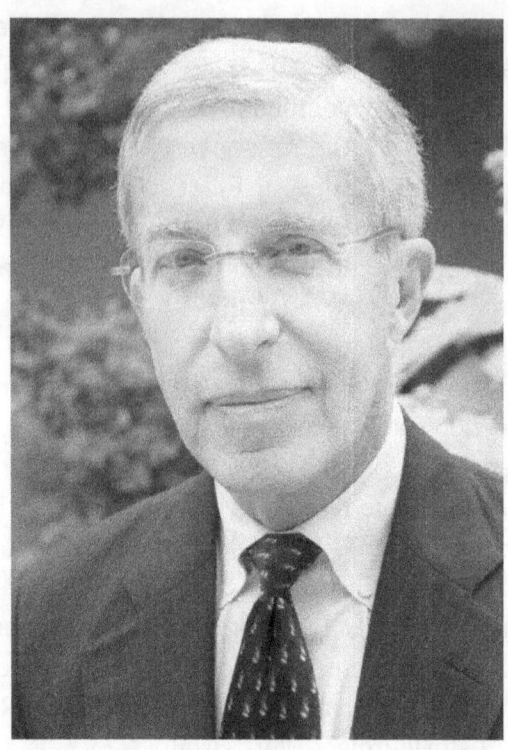

Lazar J. Greenfield, MD

Lazar J. Greenfield was born in Houston in 1934 and attended Rice University before graduating from Baylor University College of Medicine in 1958. He trained in general and thoracic surgery at Johns Hopkins Hospital from 1958 to 1966. During that time, he spent two years doing research at the NIH.

Dr. Greenfield began his academic career as an Assistant Professor of Surgery and Chief of the Surgical Service at the VA Hospital of the University of Oklahoma Medical Center in 1966. He was soon named as a Markle Scholar and later became Professor of Surgery in 1971.

In 1974, Dr. Greenfield was recruited to be Chairman of the Department of Surgery at the Medical College of Virginia Commonwealth University in Richmond, VA. He remained there until 1987 when he was appointed the F.A. Coller Professor of Surgery and Chairman of the Department of Surgery at the University of Michigan.

Dr. Greenfield is best known for the development of the vena cava filter to prevent pulmonary embolism that now bears his name and is called the Greenfield Filter. He traces his thinking about the development of the vena cava filter to a frustrating experience operating on a patient with massive pulmonary emboli. He was able to extract pulmonary thrombus, but the emboli were recurrent after the procedure.

Dr. Greenfield wanted to develop a way to extract thrombus from the pulmonary circulation that would avoid a major operation. Because of his extensive catheter experience at the NIH, he felt that putting a cup on the end of a catheter could solve the problem. This method salvaged ten patients, but often the pulmonary emboli were recurrent. Dr. Greenfield then collaborated with a petroleum engineer, who likened the problem to difficulties experienced with sludge in pipelines. Together they designed a conical device that could trap clot in the circulation and still allow flow around the filter. They actually designed a delivery system in a worker's garage. Soon trials were completed with dogs and two years later, in 1973, the Greenfield vena cava filter was available for use in humans.

Dr. Greenfield has produced more than 400 scientific articles in peer-reviewed journals as well as two major textbooks of surgery. He has received many awards including the René Leriche Award and the Jacobson Innovation Award from the American College of Surgeons. He is most proud of the annual research awards in his name that have been established at the Medical College of Virginia and at the University of Michigan.

Dr. Greenfield has been elected President of the American Association of Vascular Surgery, the American Venous Forum, the American Surgical Association and many other organizations. After many years as Surgical Chair at the University of Michigan, he retired and was appointed interim Executive Vice President for Medical Affairs and CEO of the University of Michigan Health System from 2003–2004.

Dr. Greenfield retired from the University in 2004, but he remains a consultant to the FDA and the Medical Product Surveillance network. In addition to his career as a surgeon, Dr. Greenfield has been happily married to his wife, Sharon, since 1956. They have three children and eight grandchildren.

Scan the QR code below or enter the YouTube link to watch the entire interview with Dr. Lazar J. Greenfield conducted by Peter F. Lawrence, MD, brought to you by the SVS History Project Work Group.

 http://tinyurl.com/GFieldXL

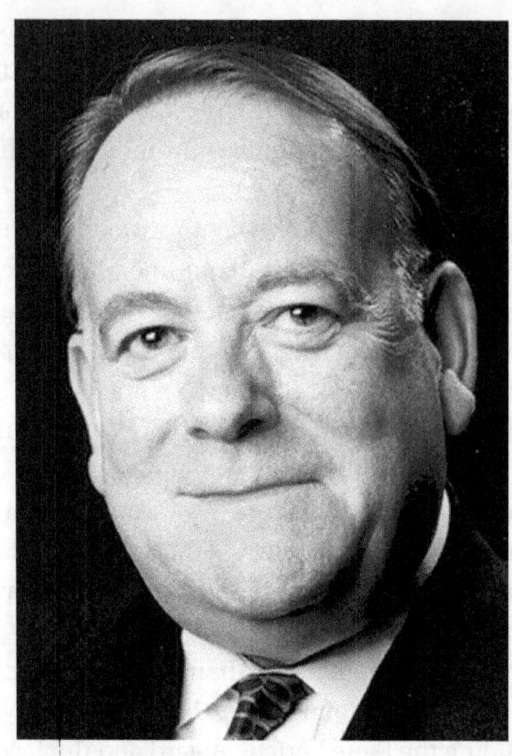

Roger M. Greenhalgh, MD

Roger Greenhalgh was born in Ilkeston, in Derbyshire, England, on February 6, 1941. His father had trained as a motor mechanic, but he worked as a policeman in Manchester. Because of World War II and the bombs falling in Manchester, Roger's family had moved to the countryside town of Ilkeston before he was born. He attended grammar school at Ilkeston.

His headmaster at Ilkeston recommended that he go into medicine, despite the engineering focus of his studies. Mr. Greenhalgh applied to and was accepted at St. Thomas' Hospital Medical School in London. There, one of the faculty, Mr. Gordon Wright told him that he should become a surgeon, which planted a valuable seed.

After surgical training at St. Thomas', he went to rotations of various specialties at Hammersmith Hospital. During this time, he found a love of vascular surgery. The pioneer vascular surgeon Professor Peter Martin inspired him by telling him that he would go on to solve problems that Mr. Martin could not.

In 1964, Mr. Greenhalgh married Karin Maria Gross, to whom he had been introduced by their two fathers years before, when he was 16 years old. While in training, in 1974, Mr. Greenhalgh won the prestigious Moynihan Fellowship of the Association of Surgeons of Great Britain and Ireland. The £1,000 stipend was to be used to visit worldwide centers of excellence.

Since his mentors, including Mr. Martin, Mr. Frank Crockett, Mr. Jerry Taylor and Mr. Felix Eastcott had all spent time abroad and had many helpful connections, Greenhalgh used his Moynihan prize to tour major vascular centers around the world and also in the U.S. from San Francisco to Boston. He was able to meet many legendary surgical leaders along the way. He credits this travel as the inspiration to found the European Society for Vascular Surgery in 1987, and also the *European Journal of Vascular Surgery*.

In 1973, he was appointed as a consultant to the new Charring Cross Hospital in London which soon became the home of the Charring Cross International Symposium. Mr. Greenhalgh had been so impressed by the John Bergan and James Yao Vascular Symposium in Chicago, that he decided to emulate it in London. He has chaired this iconic meeting, which is in its 45th year, and will welcome over 4,000 participants in 2023.

Following the advances by the North American Symptomatic Carotid Endarterectomy Trial (NASCET) for carotid surgery, Mr. Greenhalgh became particularly interested in the power of randomized trials. He became a proponent of clinical trials to generate acceptance for new treatments, thereby saving many lives. Among his many papers, he has written about the appropriateness of operating on smaller aneurysms as well as a series of follow-ups of early endovascular cases, charting their durability and striving to intervene before rupture.

Mr. Greenhalgh became deeply involved in establishing certification for vascular surgery as a specialty in Europe. Among his many leadership positions and honors he was named Honorary Life President of the European Board of Vascular Surgery. He authored over 340 papers and 36 books including his memoir, *Born to Be a Surgeon*.

Scan the QR code below or enter the YouTube link to watch the entire interview with Mr. Roger M. Greenhalgh conducted by Roger T. Gregory, MD, brought to you by the SVS History Project Work Group.

 http://tinyurl.com/GhalghXR

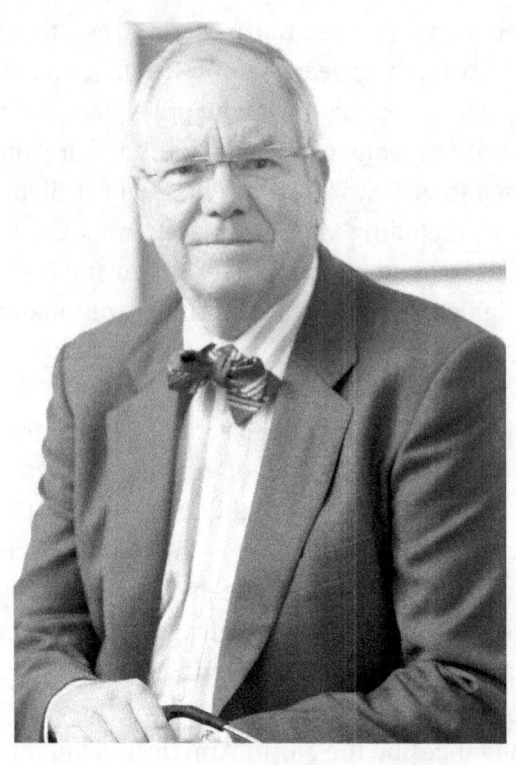

John P. Harris, MD

John Preston Harris is Emeritus Professor of Vascular Surgery at the Royal Prince Alfred Hospital in Sydney, Australia. He was born on February 21, 1949 in Grafton, New South Wales, Australia. His family background is rich with medical pedigree as his father was a general practitioner and his mother a nurse. Medicine on his father's side goes back six generations. John, who has always enjoyed working with his hands and had been introduced to woodworking by his father, combined that with an enjoyment of anatomy to decide on surgery as a career.

His Bachelor of Medicine and Bachelor of Surgery were completed in 1972 at the Saint Andrew's College, University of Sydney, where he also completed a Master of Surgery degree in 1985. He had additional surgical training at Rabaul in Papua, New Guinea and held a fellowship at Southend in England. An important part of his vascular surgery career relates to serving as the Conrad Jobst Fellow in peripheral vascular surgery at Northwestern University in

Chicago, USA. This experience, in 1980 and 1981, involved training with John J. Bergan, James S.T. Yao, and William Flinn.

Mr. Harris returned to his alma mater, Royal Prince Alfred Hospital at the University of Sydney, and eventually was appointed as the Foundation Professor in Vascular Surgery. He also served as the Chairman of the Division of Surgery from 1995 to 2014. Throughout his long clinical and teaching career he has written more than 130 peer-reviewed papers, 43 chapters and 82 editorial and review articles.

John Harris has received many honors, including being President of the Australian and New Zealand Society for Vascular Surgery, Editor-in-Chief for the *Australian New Zealand Journal of Surgery* (2011–2018), and being made Companion of the Royal Australasian College of Surgeons in 2019. He was selected as a member of the Order of Australia for "advances in vascular surgery, vascular ultrasound, medical education and healthcare administration" in 2007. He is a Distinguished Fellow of the Society for Vascular Surgery in North America, having been elected to Honorary Fellowship of that society in 2013. Mr. Harris is also an honorary member of the Society for Vascular Surgery for Great Britain and Ireland.

With his wife, Linda, they have raised three daughters and now have three grandchildren. Since retiring, Mr. Harris has had more time for playing guitar and "brushing up" on his astronomy.

Scan the QR code below or enter the YouTube link to watch the entire interview with Professor John P. Harris conducted by Melina R. Kibbe, MD, brought to you by the SVS History Project Work Group.

 http://tinyurl.com/HarrisXJ

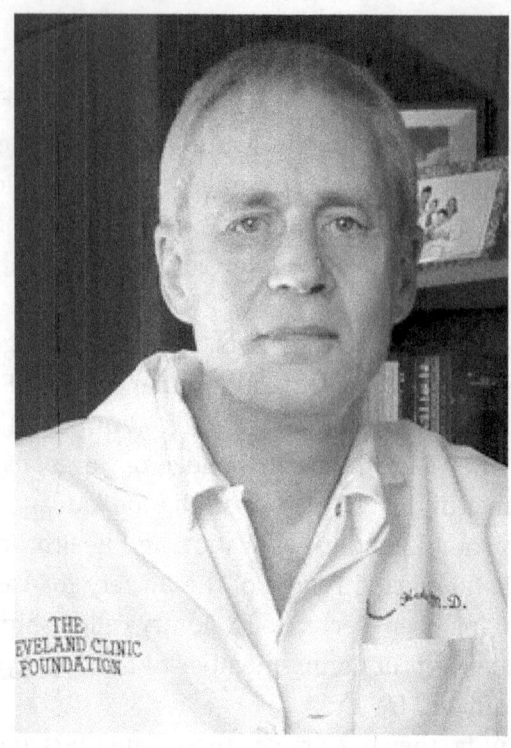

Norman R. Hertzer, MD

Norman R. Hertzer obtained his undergraduate (1964) and medical education (1967) at Indiana University where he was both Phi Beta Kappa and Alpha Omega Alpha. He was born in Toledo, Ohio, but was raised in Lafayette, Indiana, where his father worked as a salesman. Following medical school, both his general surgery residency (1967–1972) and vascular surgery fellowship (1974–1975) were at the Cleveland Clinic. He was appointed to the Clinic staff in 1976. Early on at the Cleveland Clinic he had the opportunity to be trained by and then practice with the legendary surgeons Alfred W. Humphries and Edwin G. Beven, who were the first two leaders of vascular surgery at the Clinic. Dr. Hertzer himself later became Chairman of the Department of Vascular Surgery in 1989.

Early in his career he was named as a traveling fellow of the James IV Association of Surgeons, which included a stipend with which Dr. Hertzer and his wife were able to visit numerous vascular centers in Europe. They were hosted by many pioneer vascular surgeons including Edouard Kieffer in Paris and Felix Eastcott in London. In Scotland he was even invited to golf on the Old Course in St. Andrews!

Dr. Hertzer is the author of more than 200 publications, including several articles regarding the nearly 5,000 aortic aneurysm, carotid and lower extremity procedures that he performed before retiring in 2005. One of his most important ideas was that peripheral atherosclerosis was strongly correlated with significant coronary artery plaque. He demonstrated this concept, which now seems obvious to all clinicians, in one of his landmark papers. Dr. Hertzer was a member of the Editorial Board of the *Journal of Vascular Surgery* for many years and also served as an Associate Editor.

Among his honors, Dr. Hertzer has been the Secretary and President of the Society for Vascular Surgery. He was also President of the Midwestern Vascular Surgical Society. He has received the Master Clinician (2001) and Distinguished Alumnus Awards (2003) and also the Sones/Favaloro Award (2015) from the Cleveland Clinic. He was named a Distinguished Alumnus of Indiana University in 2000.

He and his wife, Maryanne, met when they were sophomores in college and now have three children and six grandchildren.

Scan the QR code below or enter the YouTube link to watch the entire interview with Dr. Norman R. Hertzer, MD conducted by Walter J. McCarthy, MD, brought to you by the SVS History Project Work Group.

 http://tinyurl.com/HertzerXN

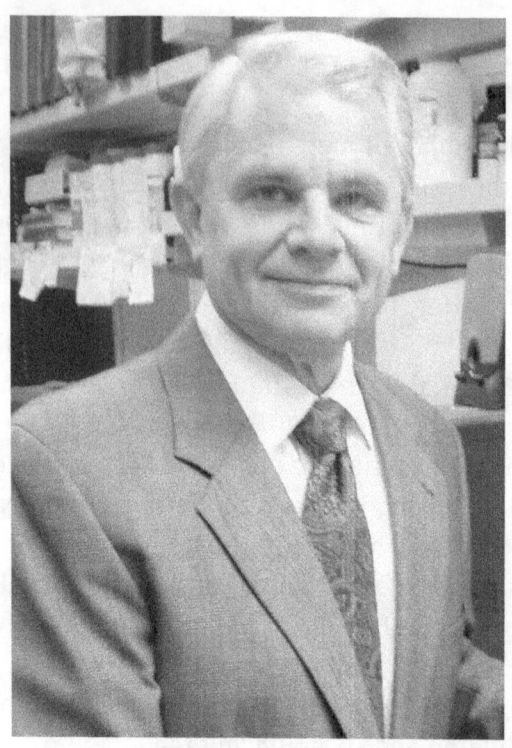

Larry H. Hollier, MD

Larry H. Hollier was born in Crowley, Louisiana on April 18, 1943. His mother was a homemaker; his father was in the hardware business and also managed a John Deere manufacturing operation. Larry traveled for college to Louisiana State University in Baton Rouge, 75 miles east of Crowley. In 1964, he married Diana Johnson with whom he has two children. He attended medical school in New Orleans at Louisiana State University and was accepted into the general surgery training program there at Charity Hospital where Isidore Cohn was the chief of surgery. He remained in surgical training from 1968 until finishing as the chief resident at Charity Hospital in 1975. During those seven years, Dr. Hollier spent two years in the United States Air Force in Maxwell, Alabama, fulfilling his military Berry Plan obligation.

He also spent one year, 1973 to 1974, at Baylor University in Dallas, Texas for a vascular surgery fellowship under renowned vascular surgeon Jesse Thompson. Dr. Cohn asked him to remain in New Orleans after his training. He soon founded the Division of Vascular Surgery and the vascular training program at Louisiana State University, directing these programs from 1975–1980.

Dr. Hollier was then recruited to the Mayo Clinic in Rochester, Minnesota, where he established the Division of Vascular Surgery and the vascular surgery training program. He was Chief of Vascular Surgery at the Mayo Clinic from 1980 until 1987. Returning to Louisiana in 1987, he became the Chairman of Surgery at the Ochsner Clinic in New Orleans and was also elected to the board of management of the Ochsner Clinic. In 1993, he accepted a unique opportunity to become Director of Clinical Affairs and Chairman of Surgery at Health Care International Medical Center in Glasgow, Scotland. This new project was envisioned to become a major referral center for Europe and the Middle East and was affiliated with Harvard Medical School and the University of Glasgow.

Dr. Hollier remained in Scotland until 1996 when he returned to the United States and was appointed Chairman of Surgery and Surgeon-in-Chief at the Mount Sinai Medical Center in New York City. In 2002, he became President and Chief Operating Officer of that institution. An opportunity came to return to Louisiana in 2004, when he was appointed Dean of the School of Medicine for Louisiana State Health Sciences Center in New Orleans and he is currently chancellor of that system.

Throughout his career, Dr. Hollier has continued to see patients, teach students, residents and surgical fellows and to perform major surgery. He has a special, career-long expertise in thoracoabdominal aneurysm repair and significant research experience documenting the efficacy of spinal fluid drainage to reduce spinal cord ischemia during those operations.

Dr. Hollier is a member of numerous surgical societies and has been a president of many. He has written more than 376 papers and chapters related to vascular surgery and medical topics.

Scan the QR code below or enter the YouTube link to watch the entire interview with Dr. Larry H. Hollier conducted by Roger T. Gregory, MD, brought to you by the SVS History Project Work Group.

 http://tinyurl.com/HollierXL

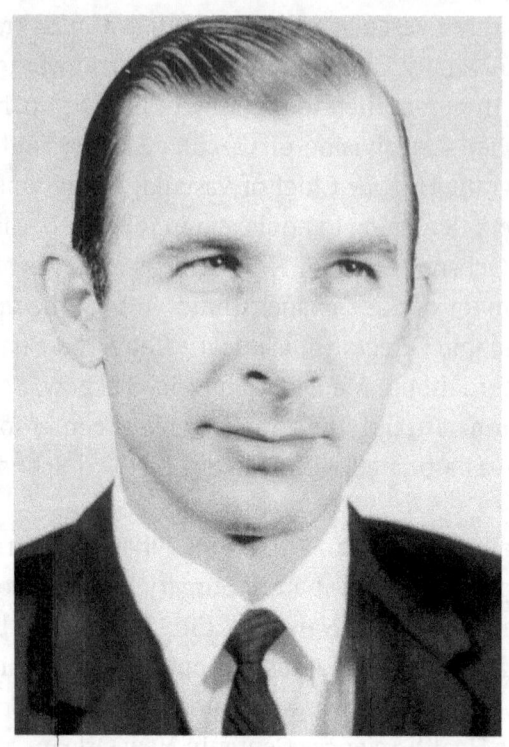

Jimmy F. Howell, MD

Jimmy F. Howell was born on September 10, 1932 in Winnfield, Louisiana. His father was a rancher and drilled oil wells. He received a BS degree in 1954 from Lamar Technological Institute, Beaumont, Texas and an MD degree in 1957 from Baylor College of Medicine in Houston, Texas. After completing his general surgical residency at Baylor, he entered the thoracic surgical residency there in 1963. He was asked to join the Baylor faculty as an Assistant Professor in 1964 by Michael DeBakey and had risen to Professor of Surgery by 1975. He served as director of the vascular surgery training programs at Baylor and the Methodist Hospital for many years.

Dr. Howell attributes his skill in peripheral vascular surgery, for which he became widely known, to Dr. DeBakey, and Drs. Stanley Crawford and George Morris. He credits Dr. Denton Cooley for teaching him his equally renowned skill as a cardiac surgeon.

Howell and H. Edward Garrett were among the first to ever perform a vein graft to the anterior tibial and posterior tibial arteries respectively. They were very familiar with using reverse saphenous vein grafts in the femoral to popliteal configuration at that time. Howell recalls the first anterior tibial bypass for a diabetic patient with first toe gangrene who had failed a lumbar sympathectomy. He decided on a lateral knee tunnel, carefully placed so the graft would not kink with knee flexion.

Inspired by his mentor and colleague, Dr. Garrett, Howell did research on coronary ischemia. In 1964, this ultimately resulted in the two of them performing the first ever coronary artery bypass operation (CAB). Their case involved a total right coronary occlusion and obstruction of the left main and proximal left coronary artery. It was performed with a reversed saphenous vein graft from the ascending aorta to the anterior descending coronary artery. The anastomosis was done with the heart beating. The patient returned seven years later for angiography and the vein graft was completely patent with a 60% stenosis at the toe and most of the flow going retrograde into the circumflex coronary artery. This spectacular event, together with the groundwork started at the Cleveland Clinic, quickly established the CAB graft as the most frequently performed heart operation.

In the extremely competitive environment of Houston, Howell emerged a master surgeon with an impeccable reputation. Recently, the *DeBakey Cardiovascular Journal* examined four decades of Dr. Howell's operative cases. In four decades, he operated on 27,632 cases excluding thoracic (pulmonary) cases. There were 3,688 carotid endarterectomy cases with a stroke and death rate of 1.05% and the rate was 0.3% for the last ten years of the review. Revascularization of the femoral, popliteal and tibial arteries was performed in 1,367 patients with a 1.0% 30-day operative mortality rate. Howell also treated a significant number of patients with thoracic or thoracoabdominal aneurysms and visceral artery occlusive disease.

Jimmy Howell was married for 60 years to Roberta Blankstein, who he met in college at Lamar. They have six children and 13 grandchildren. He was an avid outdoorsman and rancher, owning a 16,000-acre ranch with 2,000 head of cattle. Dr. Howell died on December 22, 2014.

Scan the QR code below or enter the YouTube link to watch the entire interview with Dr. Jimmy F. Howell conducted by Roger T. Gregory, MD, brought to you by the SVS History Project Work Group.

 http://tinyurl.com/HowellXJ1

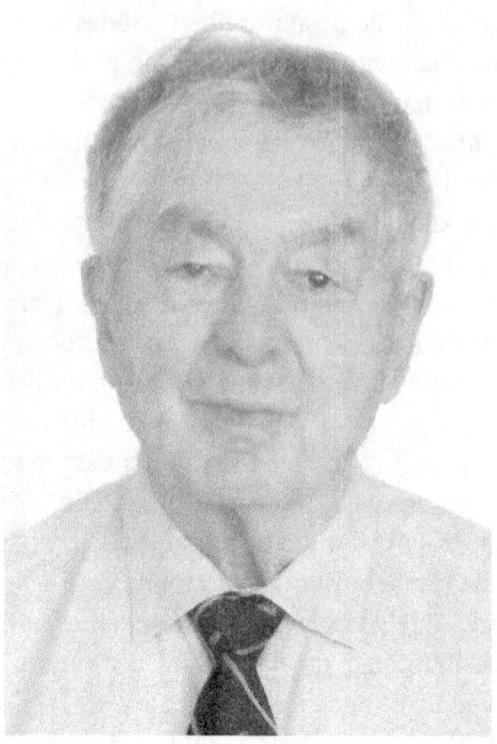

Anthony M. Imparato, MD

Anthony Imparato is a genuine New Yorker, born in Brooklyn in 1922. Tony's father, a first-generation Italian American, arranged for him to spend two years back in Italy when he was between eight and ten years old. As a result, Tony was gifted with almost perfect spoken Italian. Otherwise, his education was in the New York City public system. His BA and MD degrees were from Columbia College and then from New York University (1946), all in New York City. He then served in the Navy and at the time of his discharge found it was too late in the season to start a surgical residency. Consequently, he accepted a position for one year as an anatomy prosector and teacher.

He then progressed into clinical training on the New York University (NYU) Postgraduate School Surgical Service at Bellevue Hospital. Toward the end of training, among his group of eight residents, he was chosen to be Chief Surgical Resident at Bellevue Hospital. There, Imparato served under the tutelage of Dr. Jere Lord. Dr. Lord was performing thoracic and vascular procedures and also some cardiac operations and procedures for congenital heart disease well before cardiopulmonary bypass was available. At that time, aneurysms were being treated with external wrapping, and Dr. Lord was also known for his expertise with portacaval shunt procedures. During this time, Dr. Arthur Voorhees, a contemporary of Dr. Imparato, repaired the first abdominal aortic aneurysm using a prosthetic graft. Voorhees performed the operation on the other side of New York City, at Columbia-Presbyterian Hospital. The procedure, performed in 1953, involved a handmade tube of vinyon-N synthetic cloth and would forever change the possibilities of aortic reconstruction.

Dr. Imparato began practice at NYU in 1958. He developed a busy surgical practice, became the Chief of the Division of Vascular Surgery for over 20 years, and in 1975 became a Professor of Surgery at NYU.

In 1962 Dr. Imparato established one of the very first vascular fellowships in the country, with George Sanoudas as his first fellow. Throughout his clinical career, he taught his many fellows the importance of technical excellence. His favorite operation was the carotid endarterectomy because of the fine technique required and the sensitivity and importance of the end organ.

Dr. Imparato had a number of important insights. Many, which at the time seemed revolutionary, are now standard teaching. He was the first to suggest that exercise can relieve some of the intermittent claudication symptoms for patients with femoral popliteal artery stenosis or occlusion. His observation of hemorrhage under carotid plaque further expanded the thinking about the pathogenesis of carotid embolic symptoms. Imparato was among the first to recognize patterns of Dacron graft failure after aortic graft replacement surgery. He performed experimental surgery to better understand intimal hyperplasia and published on that topic in 1972 before any others had.

Among his many honors, Dr. Imparato was elected as the 39th President of the Society of Vascular Surgery (SVS) in 1985 and was awarded with the Distinguished Service Award from the SVS in 2003.

Dr. Imparato married Agatha Petriccione in 1943. They were married for 68 years. Dr. Imparato moved to Florida in retirement and died in St. Petersburg, Florida on February 12, 2018 at age 95.

Scan the QR code below or enter the YouTube link to watch the entire interview with Dr. Anthony M. Imparato conducted by Roger T. Gregory, MD, brought to you by the SVS History Project Work Group.

 http://tinyurl.com/ImparXA

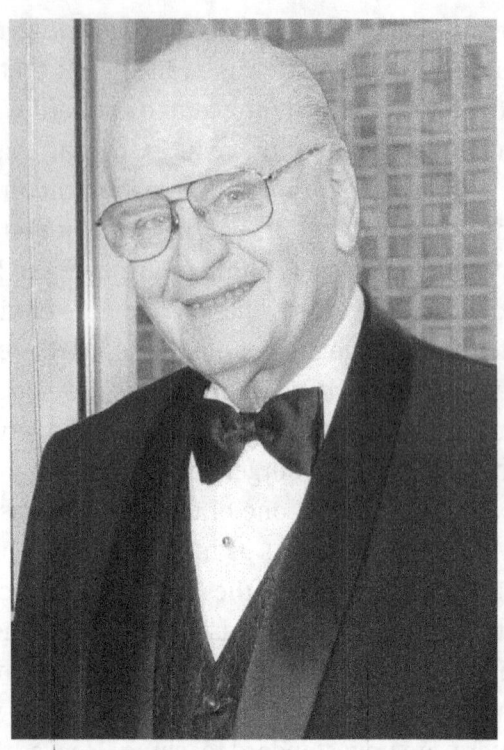

Julius H. Jacobson II, MD

Julius Jacobson is remembered as the father of microvascular surgery and also as a chief of vascular surgery at Mount Sinai Hospital in New York City. He was born in 1927 in Toledo, Ohio, his father a lawyer, and his mother a homemaker. The family moved to Detroit, to Chicago, and then permanently to Manhattan when Julius was eight years old. He was educated in the New York City public school system, and was able to attend the magnet high school called Townsend Harris. This school was taught by college professors who taught the high school students and was only a three-year curriculum. He therefore graduated when he was 15 years old. Julius, however, did not have the funds to attend college and took a job as a photographer. Eventually, he was admitted to the University of Toledo and worked through college as a photographer.

He enlisted in the U.S. Navy at the youngest possible age in 1945 because World War II was raging, but by then the war was almost over and he was soon back at college.

After college, Julius applied to medical school, but was rejected by all 23 schools to which he had applied. This, in retrospect, led to a fortuitous occurrence. The year after not being accepted into medical school, Julius took a research position at the University of Pennsylvania, which, among other things included working with the microbe paramecium. Working with the paramecium required him to learn how to use and become very familiar with a microscope. The following year, with letters of recommendation from his research work, he was accepted by multiple medical schools and chose Johns Hopkins, graduating from Hopkins in 1952. During medical school, he was a student of Alfred Blalock who became a lifelong hero. For his surgical training, he returned to New York City, to Columbia Presbyterian Hospital, and spent seven years in training, which included general and thoracic surgery.

Dr. Jacobson's insight to apply the microscope to vessel surgery came very early in his surgical attending career. He had been asked to take a new job and become assistant professor and the director of surgical research at the University of Vermont. In the animal laboratory there, some of the researchers were having considerable difficulty anastomosing small laboratory animal arteries for one of their experiments. Dr. Jacobson had the intuition, based on his previous experience with the microscope, that applying significant magnification could make these anastomoses possible. At that time, current teaching was that blood vessels less than seven mms in diameter could not be anastomosed successfully. This approach, of course, worked well, and in the years to come Dr. Jacobson went on to develop many instruments, techniques and suture applications for microvascular surgery. He recognized and taught others the importance of using the finger muscles for microsurgery rather than relying on the action of the wrist for greater delicacy. Importantly, he also worked with the Carl Zeiss microscope company in West Germany to develop an operating microscope that had a separate second pair of binocular eyepieces. This invention, which he called the "diploscope" allowed two surgeons to work together, one as an assistant, and also allowed teaching technique under the microscope. Dr. Jacobson used the original prototype clinically for years, and it is now in the Smithsonian Museum in Washington, DC.

During his long career as a vascular surgeon, including directing the vascular unit at Mount Sinai Hospital in New York City, Dr. Jacobson recalls that his favorite operations were the leg bypass operations.

Later in his life, Dr. Jacobson became a very significant philanthropist. He generously endowed five professorships of surgery at universities in the United States and also in Israel. He has made significant donations to the Society for Vascular Surgery. In addition, Dr. Jacobson and his wife, Joan, established two annual awards through the American College of Surgeons. One is an innovation award for established researcher-inventors, and the other, a promising investigator award.

Julius Jacobson passed away on December 4, 2022 at age 95.

Scan the QR code below or enter the YouTube link to watch the entire interview with Dr. Julius H. Jacobson II, conducted by Roger T. Gregory, MD, brought to you by the SVS History Project Work Group.

 http://tinyurl.com/JacobsonXJ

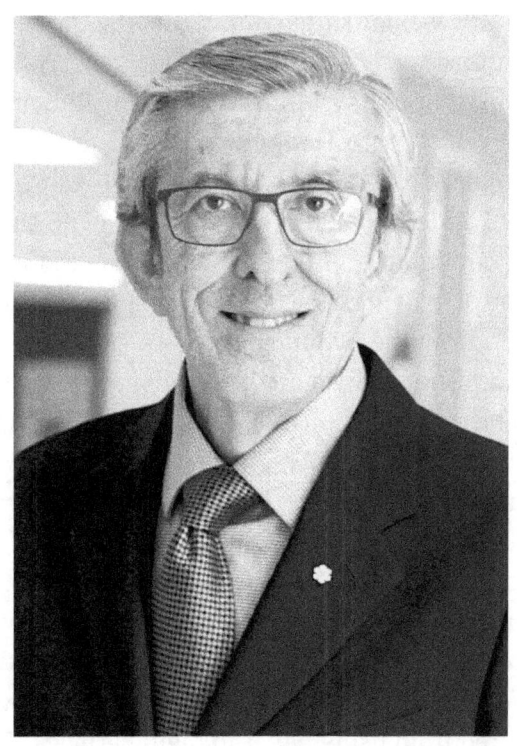

K. Wayne Johnston, MD

K. Wayne Johnston was raised, educated, and has always worked in Toronto, Canada. He was born 30 miles north of Toronto on February 22, 1943 in the town of Bradford. His father had been trained to work as an aircraft mechanic during World War II, and at the end of the war entered engineering school and became an engineer professionally. Dr. Johnston's mother was a registered nurse and always anticipated that her son would become a surgeon. Wayne was inspired by his hard-working uncle, who was a pharmacist and the only other family member to work in a medical field.

    Wayne went straight from high school into medical school at the University of Toronto. He was able to extern one summer working in a cancer clinic during medical school, where Wayne was introduced to clinical research and had his first view of life-table statistics. He married one of his medical school classmates, Jean E. Turley, who became a neurologist, and with whom he had two children. His surgical training was at the University of Toronto where he became interested in vascular surgery, intrigued by the technical challenges of doing the operations.

Dr. Johnston's vascular fellowship was with Ronald Baird and Donald Wilson at the University of Toronto. Dr. Baird was the one who introduced him to the Society for Vascular Surgery (SVS), taking him to a meeting when he was a young attending. This led to a long SVS affiliation, with Dr. Johnston serving on many different committees of the SVS over more than 25 years and eventually becoming the president of the Society in 2007. He received the Lifetime Achievement Award from the SVS in 2009.

Dr. Johnston established a division of vascular surgery at the University of Toronto in 1981 and led the division as chairman until 2003. He was chosen as a James IV Traveling Scholar in 1984, during which time he was able to travel abroad to important surgical centers. He had an extremely busy surgical practice during the 1980s and 1990s, remembering the repair of aortic aneurysms and juxta-renal aortic aneurysms as his favorite operations.

One of Dr. Johnston's most important responsibilities was serving as the co-editor of the *Journal of Vascular Surgery* with Robert Rutherford from 1996 until 2003. They directed the *Journal* during the innovative time when the publication converted from using paper to digital articles. They also initiated important conflict-of-interest and ethics guidelines for authors.

Dr. Johnston worked with Jack Cronenwett as a co-editor of *Rutherford's Textbook of Vascular Surgery*, producing the seventh edition in 2010 and the eighth edition in 2014. They supervised this extremely important textbook during the interesting time when the copyright for the book moved to the SVS through a contract with Elsevier publishing company.

Dr. Johnston has had many responsibilities within Canadian surgery including being a co-founder of the Canadian Society for Vascular Surgery in 1978 and serving as its president in 1987.

Throughout his career he has been known worldwide for innovation with ultrasound including applying that technique to blood vessel hemodynamic issues. Many of his most important ideas and papers relate to those topics. For his many contributions, K. Wayne Johnston was recognized as a member of the Order of Canada in 2018.

Scan the QR code below or enter the YouTube link to watch the entire interview with Dr. K. Wayne Johnston conducted by Norman M. Rich, MD, and Peter F. Lawrence, MD, brought to you by the SVS History Project Work Group.

 http://tinyurl.com/JohnXKW1

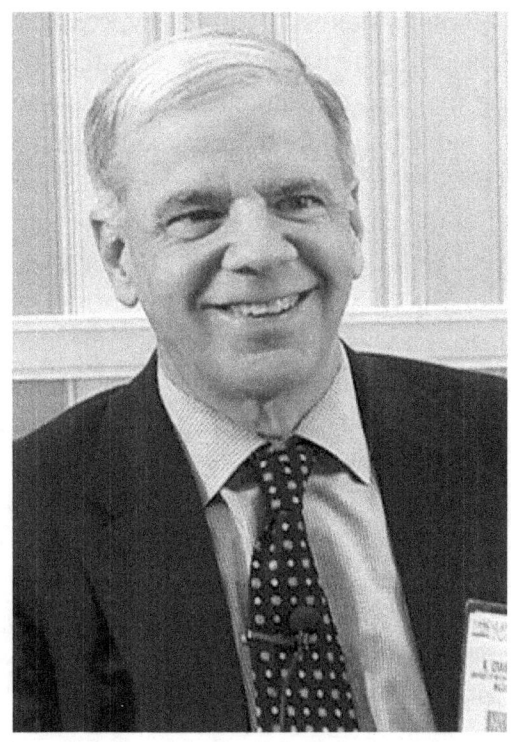

K. Craig Kent, MD

Craig Kent is an American vascular surgeon, surgical educator, medical school leader and surgical researcher. Dr. Kent was raised in Fallon, Nevada, where his father was a cattle rancher on property homesteaded in the 1880s. His mother was a teacher.

Dr. Kent was admitted to the University of Nevada-Reno as an agriculture major, but he soon opted for medicine over ranching and was admitted to medical school at the University of California, San Francisco. He stayed at the same institution for general surgical residency and had his first introduction to vascular surgery through the vascular practice of pioneer surgeons Edwin "Jack" Wiley, Ronald Stoney and William Ehrenfeld. After residency, his vascular fellowship was at the Brigham and Women's Hospital under John Mannick and Andy Whittemore. He was selected as the Society for Vascular Surgery E. J. Wylie Traveling Fellow in 1994. His first appointment after fellowship was at the Beth Israel Hospital in Boston, where he established a laboratory and continued his research interest in intimal hyperplasia and vein graft stenosis. Throughout his career he has had over 25 years of funding to continue his research into the molecular mechanisms of vascular disease. As a result of this work, he has published more than 325 papers and 65 book chapters.

Dr. Kent's distinguished career is notable for many achievements including serving as Chief of the combined divisions of vascular surgery at Cornell and Columbia in New York City (2001–2008). He then was recruited to Madison, Wisconsin to be the Chairman of Surgery at the University of Wisconsin (2008–2016). In 2016 he became Dean of the College of Medicine at Ohio State University, and in February, 2020, he was asked to become Executive Vice President for Medical Affairs at the University of Virginia and CEO of UVA Health in Charlottesville, Virginia.

Dr. Kent is a past President of the Society for Vascular Surgery (2007) and served on the American Board of Surgery from 2015 to 2019 where he became Chair in 2019.

Scan the QR code below or enter the YouTube link to watch the entire interview with Dr. K. Craig Kent conducted by Peter F. Lawrence, MD, brought to you by the SVS History Project Work Group.

 http://tinyurl.com/KentXKC1

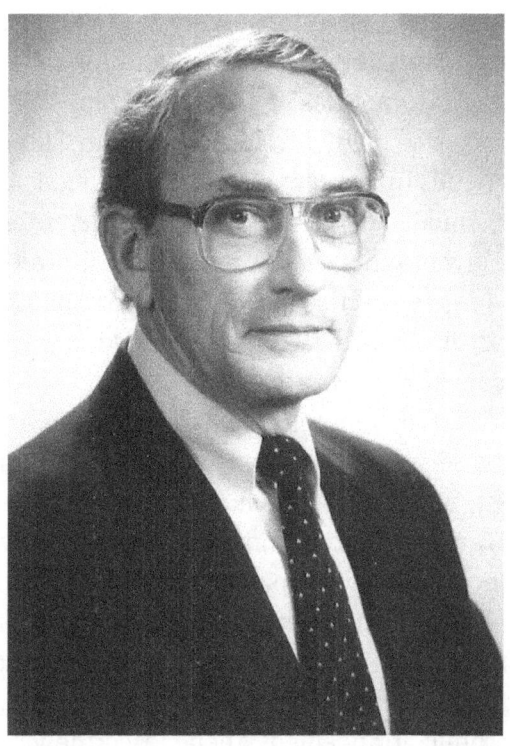

Robert L. Kistner, MD

Robert Kistner was born into a medical family in St. Louis, Missouri in 1929. His father was an ear, nose, and throat surgeon, and of the four children in the family, three became physicians. With this background, it was natural that Robert attended college at St. Louis University and then went on to medical school and general surgical training there as well.

In general surgery training, Dr. Kistner spent a great deal of time operating with C. Rollins Hanlon, who had come to be the Chairman of Surgery at St. Louis University in 1950. Dr. Hanlon had been trained by Alfred Blalock at Johns Hopkins and became a pioneer of cardiac and vascular surgery. As a resident, Dr. Kistner scrubbed with Dr. Hanlon when they performed the first prosthetic, aortic aneurysm repair in St. Louis using a homemade prosthetic graft in 1953. Dr. Hanlon became a lifelong role model for Dr. Kistner.

Following surgical training, Dr. Kistner spent two years in the Air Force and then practiced general surgery in Santa Barbara, California. He was given the opportunity to be trained in vascular surgery at the Cleveland Clinic in 1964. He accepted a one-and-a-half-year position working under the vascular surgery pioneers there, Al Humphries and Edwin Bevan.

In 1966, Dr. Kistner was invited to join the Straub Clinic in Honolulu, Hawaii by one of his friends from general surgery training. For the rest of his professional life he remained in Honolulu, with an academic association through the University of Hawaii where he became clinical professor of surgery in 1986. His vascular surgery practice in Honolulu was mainly related to arterial disease, but he soon also became deeply interested in the largely unresolved problem of venous insufficiency.

Soon after his arrival in Honolulu, he performed the first case of deep venous valve repair by re-suspension. He is now known worldwide for this operation. The patient, an electrical lineman, had had an electrical injury and venous thrombosis, and was left with an incapacitating leg swelling. Ascending and descending venograms showed patent deep veins in the thigh without any functioning valve closure. Dr. Kistner decided to surgically explore the femoral vein just distal to the common femoral vein. On opening that vessel he found a very relaxed, redundant set of valve leaflets. He re-suspended the valve with suture into an anatomic arrangement, then closed the vein. Almost immediately the patient noticed extreme improvement in his leg swelling symptoms. The patient did well, living for 13 more years. This led to a published clinical report in 1968 and many, many more surgical repairs over the following years.

Spurred by the lack of organization in reporting venous disease, Dr. Kistner was involved with developing the system used today. Working with his partner, Bo Eklöf, he spearheaded a symposium in Hawaii sponsored by the American Venous Forum that initiated the first practical way of categorizing lower-extremity venous insufficiency. An international meeting of experts in 1994 established the CEAP (clinical, etiologic, anatomical, physiologic) system. This system is still widely used by practitioners.

Scan the QR code below or enter the YouTube link to watch the entire interview with Dr. Robert L Kistner conducted by Walter J. McCarthy, MD, brought to you by the SVS History Project Work Group.

 http://tinyurl.com/KistnerXR

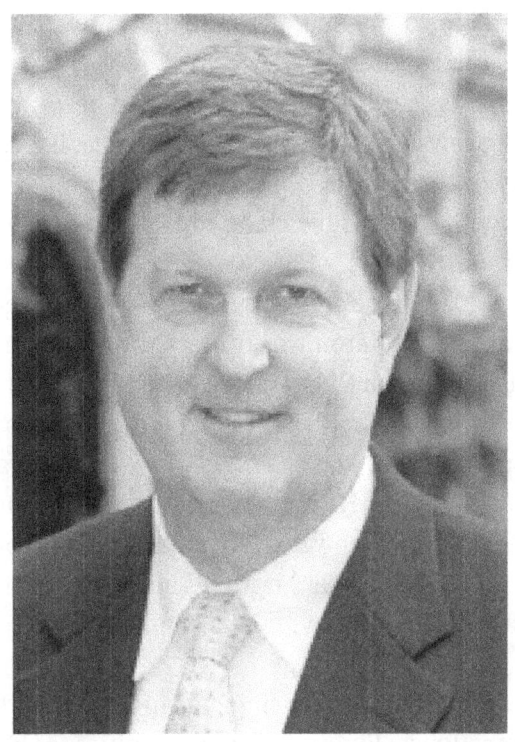

Peter F. Lawrence, MD

Peter Lawrence grew up in Haddonfield, a town in southwest New Jersey, which is a suburb of Philadelphia. The family lived on a six-acre rural property, where his father, an electrical engineer, built their home. His father worked in nearby Camden for the Radio Corporation of America (RCA).

Besides his usual studies, Peter remembers spending a great deal of time with his father on woodworking projects, including building wooden boats in the basement, and also refinishing and restoring boats. In high school, he learned to be a very good small-boat sailor and was involved with championship racing in Laser-class sailboats.

Peter was an excellent high school athlete, and this continued at Dartmouth College where he was an outstanding defensive end in football and a lacrosse player. He ended up receiving several college all-star athletic awards. He was invited to try out for the Dallas Cowboys and the Denver Broncos, but this was interrupted by a serious shoulder dislocation that occurred during a rugby match. He considers this a blessing directing him toward a career in surgery rather than professional sports!

Dr. Lawrence reflects that he was lucky to have been accepted to medical school after having been so focused on sports during college. He attended Dartmouth Medical School, which was a two-year program at the time. He then transferred, along with most of his class, to Harvard Medical School to complete his third and fourth years.

Dr. Lawrence met his wife, Karen, while they were college students. When he finished medical school, Karen was in New York City doing graduate work. Thus, Peter decided to pursue general surgery training at Columbia rather than staying in Boston. His vascular surgery fellowship was also at Columbia. At that time, Arthur Voorhees was the chief of vascular surgery, and Dr. Lawrence came to know him well. He remembers housesitting on many occasions when Dr. Voorhees was away on vacation and the stories told of the very first prosthetic bypass graft—which Dr. Voorhees had pioneered in February, 1953. (This first graft was done with vinyon-N, a synthetic fabric developed during World War II.)

By 1978, Karen Lawrence was a rising star in academic literature, particularly regarding James Joyce. Finding job opportunities for both of them in Salt Lake City at the University of Utah, the couple moved west. Dr. Lawrence was appointed the chief of vascular surgery at the University of Utah, and he eventually became the chief of surgery at the VA there. During his years in Salt Lake City, Dr. Lawrence greatly enhanced the program, hiring talented young surgical faculty, developing research and also expanding the noninvasive vascular laboratory. After 20 years in Salt Lake City Dr. Lawrence moved to UC Irvine in 1998 to become the associate dean for clinical affairs. Several years later in 2003, he moved to UCLA to become the chief of vascular surgery.

Dr. Lawrence has always been very interested in teaching and relates this to his past experience teaching sailing and having been mentored by many excellent surgical teachers. He has edited two textbooks of surgery for medical students. Both books have been re-published in multiple editions and are used by most United States and international medical students. Likewise, in his roles as president of many important surgical societies he relates his successful leadership to his experience in athletics working as a team player. He was the president of the Society for Vascular Surgery from 2014 to 2015. He then served as president of the Society for Vascular Surgery Research Foundation from 2015 to 2016. Most recently, Dr. Lawrence has completed six years as co-editor of the *Journal of Vascular Surgery* with his friend and colleague, Peter Gloviczki.

Peter and Karen Lawrence have been married for many years and have two sons, Andy and Jeff. Karen was recently the president of Sarah Lawrence College outside of New York City, and is currently the president of the Huntington Library in San Marino, California.

Scan the QR code below or enter the YouTube link to watch the entire interview with Dr. Peter F. Lawrence conducted by Walter J. McCarthy, MD, William H. Pearce, MD, and James S.T. Yao, MD, brought to you by the SVS History Project Work Group.

 http://tinyurl.com/LawrenceXP

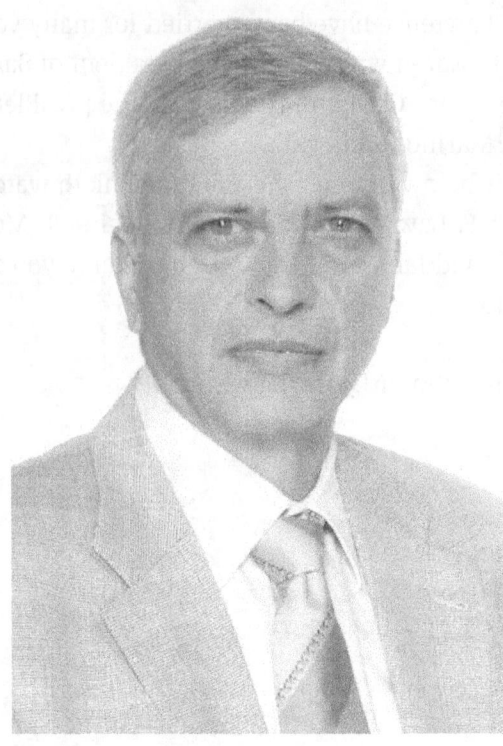

Christos D. Liapis, MD

Christos Liapis was born and raised in a beautiful and unique region of central Greece. His hometown of Kalabaka is in the foothills of the famous rocks of Meteora. These rise thousands of feet above the town with Eastern Orthodox monasteries built on their summits. His father was a general practitioner, the only physician in the region. Christos was born on February 13, 1947. World War II had just ended, and their town was still badly damaged.

His father had a huge practice that included surgery. At times, Christos accompanied his father for house calls, and sometimes they had to travel by mule to see patients in remote areas. Impressed by his father's skill, dedication and also his respected position in their town, Christos soon had decided that he would pursue medicine himself.

This decision eventually led him to medical school at the National Kapodistrian University of Athens where he also completed his general surgery residency. His father had attended the same medical school. One of his surgical mentors helped Christos decide between vascular and cardiac surgery as a career. He was told that because he had an independent spirit, he should go into vascular surgery, where he could make the diagnosis, manage the non-invasive laboratory, perform the appropriate surgery, and follow up all of his patients himself.

After general surgery residency, Dr. Liapis had the opportunity to spend three years at Ohio State University, working directly under the pioneer vascular surgeon Bill Evans. As a fellow under Dr. Evans' guidance, he produced a paper on cranial nerve injury and carotid surgery, which he presented at the Society for Vascular Surgery in Chicago in 1980. His professional and technical instruction from Dr. Evans greatly influenced his career. He also spent one additional year doing vascular research at the Massachusetts General Hospital before returning home to eventually become the Chairman of Vascular Surgery at his medical school in Athens.

In Athens he followed an extraordinarily productive career path. Dr. Liapis established the international post graduate course, "Endovascular Techniques," at the Attikon University Hospital. He recalls that his senior vascular surgeon colleague in Athens, Panagiotis Balas, truly opened the door to international relations for him. He eventually served as president of the European Society for Vascular Surgery from 2004 to 2005. He also served as president of the International Society for Vascular Surgery from 2012 to 2014.

Throughout his career, he has remained dedicated to innovative ways to teach younger surgeons, including those from abroad. His areas of research include carotid and aortic pathophysiology and experimental atherosclerosis. Dr. Liapis is the chief editor of two international textbooks and the author of more than 37 book chapters and more than 320 scientific publications.

Scan the QR code below or enter the YouTube link to watch the entire interview with Dr. Christos D. Liapis conducted by Norman M. Rich, MD, and James S.T. Yao, MD, brought to you by the SVS History Project Work Group.

 http://tinyurl.com/LiapisXC

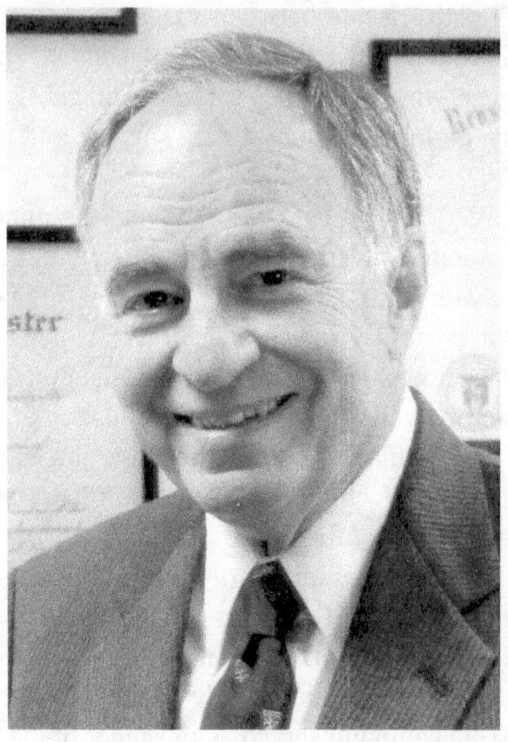

Frank W. LoGerfo, MD

Frank LoGerfo is a Boston surgeon who served as Chief of the Division of Vascular Surgery at the Beth Israel Deaconess Hospital from 1987 to 2005 and also as Chief of Surgery there from 1999 to 2001. He is well known as a skilled clinical surgeon, program director for vascular surgery and a highly successful basic science researcher.

Frank William LoGerfo was born on September 15, 1940 in Middletown, New York. His mother was a homemaker and father was a farmer who became involved in his own manufacturing business. Originally interested in engineering, Frank attended Rensselaer Polytechnic Institute but eventually became a biology major and graduated in 1962. He attended medical school at the University of Rochester School of Medicine and planned to pursue a career in research. At Rochester, he was inspired by several surgeons: Seymour Schwartz and two pioneering vascular surgeons, Charles Rob and James DeWeese.

His general surgery training was at Boston University. Dr. LoGerfo attributes much of what he knows about clinical vascular surgery to his long-time mentor, John Mannick. Later, Dr. LoGerfo founded the vascular fellowship at Boston University. His career-long interest in training surgeons included serving as the President of the Program Directors in Vascular Surgery. He also served as the Chair of the Vascular Surgery Board for the American Board of Surgery.

Dr. LoGerfo has been a researcher funded by multiple NIH grants for most of his career, including one R01 grant that was sustained for more than 33 years. He has also held funding through T32 grants for surgical residents and T35 grants for medical students. Through those grants he has trained and mentored many dozens of successful vascular surgeons and researchers.

Much of Dr. LoGerfo's research has corresponded to his long clinical interest in lower extremity ischemia, particularly in diabetic patients. It includes the analysis of flow disturbances in bypass anastomoses and the basic understanding of intimal hyperplasia at a molecular level. He has also contributed to the understanding of diabetic microcirculation and diabetic neuropathy. Celebrating his many contributions to vascular surgery, in 2013, Frank LoGerfo was awarded a Lifetime Achievement Award by the Society for Vascular Surgery.

Scan the QR code below or enter the YouTube link to watch the entire interview with Dr. Frank W. LoGerfo conducted by Norman M. Rich, MD, brought to you by the SVS History Project Work Group.

 http://tinyurl.com/LoGerfoXF

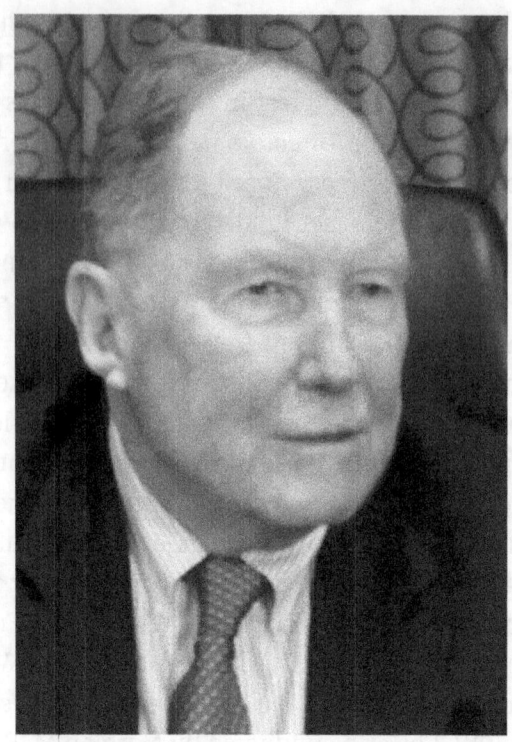

William T. Maloney

William Maloney is the only non-vascular surgeon included in this collection because of his key importance in advancing the affairs of the Society for Vascular Surgery. Mr. Maloney, with his company called Public Relations Institute (PRI), became the Executive Director for the Society for Vascular Surgery in 1974. He directed the national meeting for the first time at the annual meeting in Albuquerque, New Mexico. Previously, the Society's management had been completely handled by the SVS officers. This included contracting with hotels, selecting menus, producing programs and handling all financing. Although it is hard to imagine today, before that time it was common practice for medical societies not to have any professional management. Dr. Allan Callow is responsible for recruiting Mr. Maloney, having known him through Mr. Maloney's management of the New England Surgical Society and the Massachusetts chapter of the American College of Surgeons.

Once involved, Mr. Maloney functioned as a general advisor, facilitator of logistics, friend and confidant, and financial consultant for the Society and its officers over many years. He provided wise counsel in many areas as the Society became larger and more complicated.

Mr. Maloney participated during the development of the *Journal of Vascular Surgery* (JVS) which was first published in 1984. His positive experience using the publisher, Mosby, for other society journals helped to direct the JVS toward that publisher. Mr. Maloney also advised the Society concerning the formation of the American Venous Forum as a separate society. He was present for the deliberations related to establishing an American Board of Vascular Surgery that would be completely separate from the American Board of Surgery. The final decision to form a separate board was actually made by the senior surgeons who were involved at the Admiral's Club of O'Hare Airport in Chicago. Mr. Maloney was the one who telephoned the lawyer, Tom Rhodes, in Atlanta to draw up the papers of incorporation for the new board. This new "Vascular Board," however, was later disavowed by the American Board of Medical Specialties.

As the Society for Vascular Surgery and its sister society, the International Society for Cardiovascular Surgery (ISCVS), gained increased membership, there was a decision to obtain full-time administrative support. Mr. Maloney's tenure ended and Rebecca Maron was hired in July, 2003 as the first full-time executive director for the Society. Ms. Maron continued as director until May, 2016 and was followed in that position by Mr. Kenneth Slaw.

Mr. Maloney was born in Cambridge, Massachusetts in 1934 and passed away in 2022 at the age of 88. He graduated from Harvard College in 1955 after having taken off time during school to serve in the Army during the Korean War. After college, he joined his father's public relations company and managed PRI until he retired at age 85. He advised numerous medical and surgical societies and planned countless national and international meetings over the years. He always lived in Massachusetts, in the town of Manchester-by-the-Sea, and raised two children with Marina, his wife of 55 years.

Scan the QR code below or enter the YouTube link to watch the entire interview with William T. Maloney conducted by Norman M. Rich, MD, James S.T. Yao, MD, Jerry Goldstone, MD, Roger T. Gregory, MD, and Jonathan B. Towne, MD, brought to you by the SVS History Project Work Group.

 http://tinyurl.com/MaloneyXW

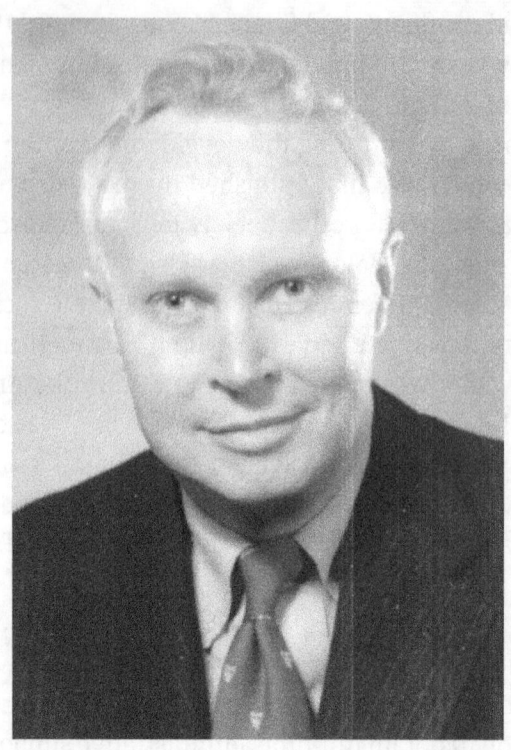

John A. Mannick, MD

John Mannick was born in Deadwood, South Dakota in 1928, but his family moved to Yakima, Washington when he was two. John's mother was a teacher, and his father was a civil engineer who had been hired to develop irrigation systems in the Yakima region. The area at that time was extremely rural. John attended public school and played varsity tennis in high school. He graduated as the class valedictorian and was offered a full scholarship to Harvard College in Boston. But John was born on March 24, 1928, meaning he was 18 at high school graduation—just old enough to join the U.S. Army. Fortunately, World War II ended in 1945, and he remembers being in the service for only six weeks!

At Harvard College, he majored in history and literature and met his wife Virginia, who was a student at Radcliffe. They married in 1952, when John was attending Harvard Medical School. Together they raised three daughters, two of whom became physicians and one a lawyer. Altogether there are seven grandchildren.

In medical school, although John had initially planned to become a psychiatrist, he found that his favorite experience was dog surgery, so he selected surgery as a specialty. He received his surgical training at the Massachusetts General Hospital, and the year that he was an intern, Michael DeBakey was the acting chief of surgery, and his chief resident was Stanley Crawford. During residency Mannick was required to fulfill the remainder of his military obligation, and he spent two years as an Air Force flight surgeon. This included learning to fly interesting aircraft, among them jet fighter training planes.

During his surgical residency, Dr. Mannick became very interested in the then theoretical idea of solid organ transplant. He elected to spend one year (1958–59) with E. Donnall Thomas working in a research lab in Cooperstown, New York. Dr. Thomas' laboratory was conducting bone marrow transplant in dogs using radiation for immuno-suppression. Thirty years later, Dr. Thomas received the 1990 Nobel Prize for his fundamental work with bone marrow transplant, sharing the prize with Joseph E. Murray and his work with kidney transplantation.

Dr. Mannick's early experience with transplantation basic science proved truly pivotal. All of his early career research was based on transplant and immune-system physiology. Later, he studied the same mechanisms in injury models. This fundamental foundation allowed continuous federal funding for his entire career up until his retirement at age 80. Of his more than 400 career publications, many of the most important contributions are based on immunology. Dr. Mannick was honored by the Society of University Surgeons with a Lifetime Achievement Award for this body of work.

His research experience also led to his first job, which was with the pioneer transplant surgeon David Hume at the Medical College of Virginia. Dr. Hume directed Dr. Mannick to focus on vascular surgery as a career path. Soon Dr. Mannick moved back to Boston University where he eventually became the Surgicial Chairman in 1973. He moved to the Brigham Hospital in 1976 to be the Surgeon-in-Chief, and from then on, he confined his clinical activities strictly to vascular surgery. During his leadership at the Brigham Hospital, Dr. Mannick expanded the department by increasing the number of full-time faculty from 20 to 62 surgeons and the number of annual surgical procedures from 8,000 to 28,000.

Throughout his career, Dr. Mannick was very interested in the vexing problem of lower-extremity ischemia. Based on his training at the Massachusetts General Hospital under Dr. Robert Linton, he became a proponent of meticulous technique using saphenous vein grafts. Dr. Mannick was performing tibial bypasses in 1961 and is among the first surgeons to ever perform an anterior tibial or peroneal artery bypass. These early operations were documented in a paper published in the journal *Surgery* in 1964. He also conceived the idea of vein bypassing to an isolated, popliteal artery segment, and published that concept in 1967.

Because of his many leadership and managerial skills, Dr. Mannick was honored as the president of many important surgical societies, including the American Surgical Association. He was also president of two American national vascular societies, the Society for Vascular Surgery from 1980 to 1981 and the International Society for Cardiovascular Surgery from 1990 to 1991. Because of his own lifelong dedication to surgical research, he was instrumental in aligning the NIH with the Society for Vascular Surgery to enhance vascular surgery research funding. As the president of The Lifeline Foundation (the Society for Vascular Surgery research foundation) he was instrumental in obtaining large amounts of funding from generous individuals, including Julius Jacobson, Thomas Fogarty, and William von Liebig.

Dr. Mannick passed away on October 13, 2019 at age 91.

Scan the QR code below or enter the YouTube link to watch the entire interview with Dr. John A. Mannick conducted by Roger T. Gregory, MD, James S.T. Yao, MD, and Walter J. McCarthy, MD, brought to you by the SVS History Project Work Group.

 http://tinyurl.com/MannickXJ

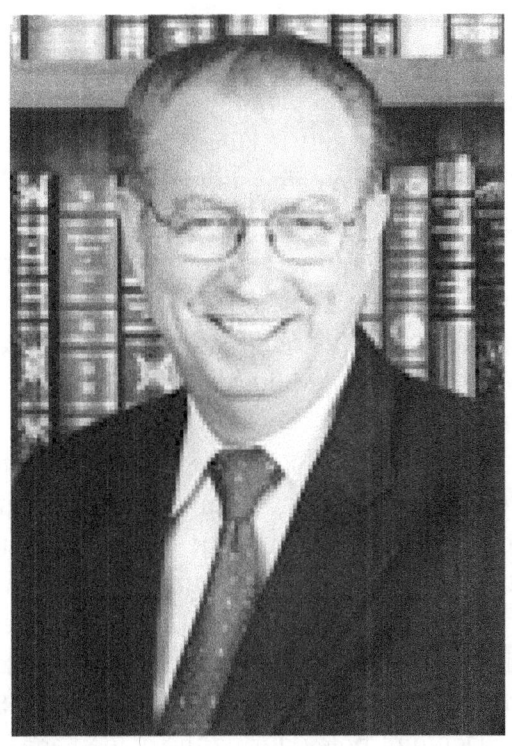

Kenneth L. Mattox, MD

Kenneth Mattox was born in White Oak, Arkansas in 1938. At that time White Oak was a town of 16 people where his father worked "choppin' cotton." When Kenneth was six months old, the family moved, traveling throughout the Southwest and southern California working as migratory farm workers. Kenneth attended grammar school in El Paso, Texas, and high school in Clovis, New Mexico. He attended Wayland Baptist College, 90 miles east of Clovis, in the Texas panhandle town of Plainview. Kenneth was the first person from either side of his family to attend college. He started out on a ministerial and music scholarship, planning to become a Baptist preacher. However, he ended up discovering a love of science instead.

Therefore, after Wayland, Dr. Mattox applied to medical school and was admitted to the Baylor College of Medicine, which he selected because it seemed to be the most competitive of all the schools that he had visited. This was consistent with his lifelong philosophy of taking the highest, hardest road. Following graduation from Baylor in 1964, Dr. Mattox completed an internship at Ben Taub Hospital in Houston, after which he needed to fulfill a two-year military obligation. He was assigned to the Aviation Accident Research Center at Fort Rucker, in Alabama. This eventually led to his first academic paper, which was related to helicopter accidents. A career-long relationship with the military ensued, related to safety equipment and survival kits for pilots as well as resuscitation and evacuation techniques. He has worked for the military on helmet design, Nomex flame-retardant flight suits, which are now also used by race-car drivers, and burn issues. This relationship lasted through the Gulf Wars, and he was awarded the Order of Military Medical Merit by the U.S. Army for his many contributions.

Dr. Mattox returned to Baylor to complete his surgical and thoracic residencies after leaving the Army. He was on hand as a young surgeon during the dynamic era of the 1960s and 1970s at the Texas Medical Center when remarkable innovations came about in vascular, cardiac, trauma and critical care surgery. He worked very closely with Dr. Michael DeBakey, absorbing many lessons while watching him in action. Dr. Mattox also had the opportunity to learn from doctors George Jordan, Arthur Beall, Stanley Crawford, George Morris and Denton Cooley during the golden age of the Texas Medical Center. He recalls that during those years Houston was "the center of the medical universe."

After Dr. Mattox completed his thoracic training, Dr. DeBakey offered him two possible jobs: He could either run one of the major ORs at Methodist Hospital or take over the surgical service at the Ben Taub Hospital, Houston's main trauma and charity hospital. Seeking a challenge, he returned to Ben Taub Hospital to direct the surgical service and later took on many important administrative roles at the hospital as well. Dr. Mattox served as the Chief of Staff at Ben Taub until 2020, when he retired after more than 40 years. His Ben Taub career choice was fundamental to him becoming the world-renowned trauma surgeon for which he is known.

Dr. Mattox is a prolific, multi-faceted writer. He is co-author of the *Trauma* textbook, now in its 9th edition, the classic Norman Rich textbook, *Vascular Trauma*, as well as the *Sabiston Textbook of General Surgery*, in its 20th edition. In addition, he wrote *Top Knife*, a book about trauma surgery, and also *The History of Surgery in Houston*. In all, he has authored more than 15 books and 600 papers. He strongly believes in communicating in a comprehensible, conversational style and in the importance of his written work as a tool to relay useful skills to other surgeons.

Dr. Mattox began his involvement with the American Association for the

Surgery of Trauma many years ago and served as president in 1995–1996. He expanded the scope of the organization by including war-zone trauma surgeons and students and residents. He has also served as president of the Texas as well as the Houston Surgical Societies. Among his many honors, in 2020, the Mathematics and Science Department at his alma mater, Wayland Baptist University, was named after him. Dr. Mattox has long been married to his wife, June, who was once the head nurse on the pediatric unit at MD Anderson. They have one daughter.

Scan the QR code below or enter the YouTube link to watch the entire interview with Dr. Kenneth L. Mattox conducted by Roger T. Gregory, MD, and James S.T. Yao, MD, brought to you by the SVS History Project Work Group.

 http://tinyurl.com/MattoxXK

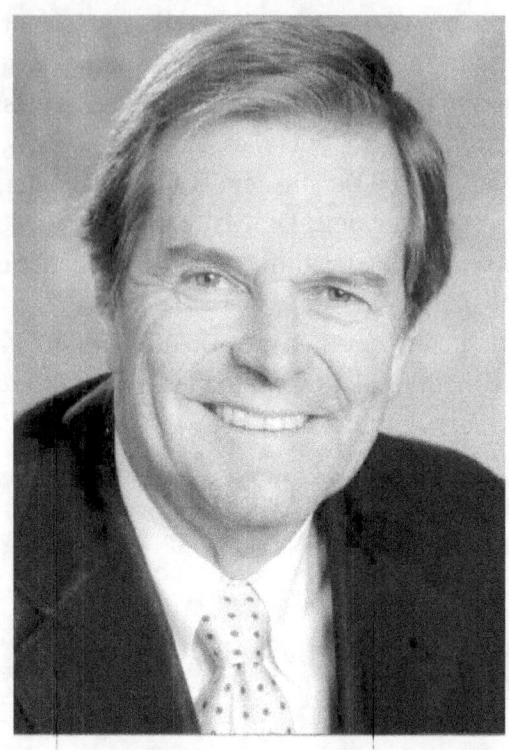

James May, MD

Professor May was the Bosch Professor of Surgery at the University of Sydney from 1979 until 2014. He also served as head of the Division of Surgery at the Royal Prince Alfred Hospital from 1979 to 1995. He was President of the Australian and New Zealand chapter of the International Society for Cardiovascular Surgery from 2001 to 2004 and the International Society of Endovascular Specialists from 2005 to 2007.

Professor May was a graduate of the University of Sydney and completed his general surgical residency at the Royal Prince Alfred Hospital in Sydney. He undertook two years of post-graduate training at the University of California, San Francisco, and the University of Manchester in the United Kingdom.

His clinical experience encompassed all aspects of vascular intervention, and his clinical research centered on endovascular treatment of aneurysms. He contributed more than 400 publications to the surgical literature, mostly related to vascular and endovascular surgery. Professor May was appointed a

Companion of the Order of Australia in 2001, his country's highest honor, for services to advance the endovascular treatment of arterial disease. He was also elected to be an Honorary Fellow of the American Surgical Association, the Society for Vascular Surgery, the Canadian Society for Vascular Surgery, the Los Angeles Surgical Society, the Asian Surgical Association and the Edward B. Diethrich Vascular Surgical Society.

Professor May was originally the only Australian to be appointed to the editorial board of the *Journal of Vascular Surgery* and was designated a Distinguished Reviewer by the editors of the JVS in 2007. He has served on the editorial boards of many other journals including the *Journal of Endovascular Therapy, Cardiovascular Surgery* and the *Journal of Vascular Diseases*.

Over his long career Professor May taught surgical trainees of every level and also medical students. In 2004, with Professor John Harris he established the Master of Surgery-by-Coursework Program, which has become a major component of surgical trainees' preparation for their practice. In retirement he continued to teach problem-based tutorials to first- and second-year medical students.

Professor May is credited with introducing endovascular surgery in Australia. His colleagues consider him the "father of vascular surgery" in the country. Born in 1934, James May passed away on March 24, 2021.

Scan the QR code below or enter the YouTube link to watch the entire interview with Dr. James May conducted by Roger T. Gregory, MD, and Peter F. Lawrence, MD, brought to you by the SVS History Project Work Group.

 http://tinyurl.com/MayXJ

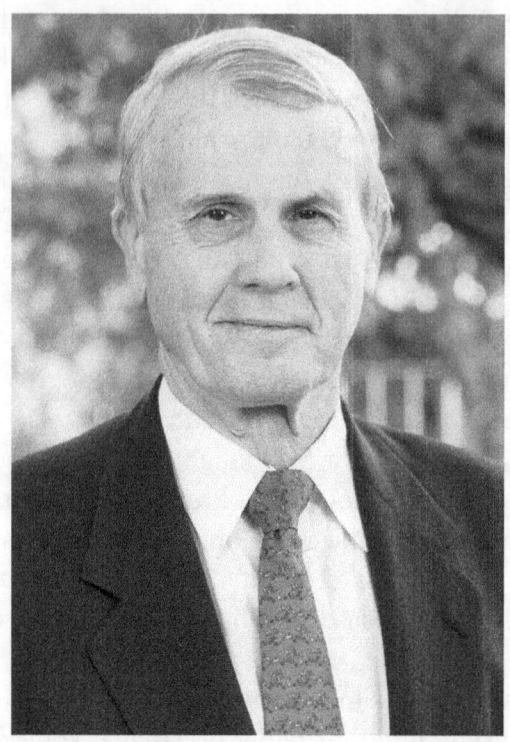

D. Craig Miller, MD

D. Craig Miller was born on December 3, 1946 in San Francisco and was raised on a working cattle ranch in the northern California mountains near Redding. After attending public high school, he was accepted to Dartmouth College, graduated in 1968, and then for medical school in 1972 returned to California to attend Stanford. His surgical and fellowship training were all there, and he has remained associated with the university for his entire career.

He is currently the Thelma and Henry Doelger Professor of Cardiovascular Surgery at the Stanford University School of Medicine. With boards in both vascular surgery and cardiothoracic surgery, Dr. Miller developed an early interest in endovascular aneurysm treatment.

With radiologist Dr. Michael Dake, the two performed one of the first endovascular stentgraft thoracic aneurysm repairs in 1992. The team used a homemade device with large Palmaz stents sewn with Prolene suture to a Cooley woven Dacron tube graft for the landmark procedure. This included ironing out the crimps in the graft fabric to decrease the graft's profile when it was being constructed the night before the operation.

Dr. Miller has a special interest in all types of aortic disease and surgery including aortic dissection, aortic valve-sparing ascending aortic repair and also mitral valve repair.

Dr. Miller's surgical training at Stanford was under the aegis of Dr. Norman Shumway in general, vascular and cardiac surgery. Dr. Shumway is well known for having performed the first human heart transplant at Stanford in 1968. Dr. Miller attributes much of his early training to the surgeons Pat Daily and Thomas Fogarty and considers Fogarty a lifelong role model.

Dr. Miller served as the program director of the vascular fellowship at Stanford from 1985 until 1993 when Chris Zarins was recruited and assumed that position. Among his many honors and responsibilities Dr. Miller is a past president of the American Association for Thoracic Surgery (2007–2008) and the Western Thoracic Surgical Association (1994–1995) and is former chairman of the American Heart Association's (AHA) Cardiovascular Surgery Council. He has received the AHA Eugene Braunwald Mentorship Award (2009), was designated a Distinguished Scientist of the American Heart Association (2003), and was a William W. L. Glenn Lecturer (2002) as well as receiving the Antoine Marfan Award (National Marfan Foundation), the Wilfred Bigelow Award (Canadian Cardiovascular Society) and the Distinguished Achievement Award (American Heart Association Cardiovascular Surgery and Anesthesia Council). Dr. Miller served as the Associate Editor for Acquired Heart Disease for *The Journal of Thoracic and Cardiovascular Surgery* for ten years.

He has been the principle investigator of NIH R01 research grants for over 30 years and has contributed more than 650 papers to the medical literature. Dr. Miller's basic and clinical research contributions have refined our understanding of mitral and aortic valve function, thoracic aortic diseases, cardiac valvular pathophysiology and ventricular mechanics. However, he believes his most rewarding accomplishments have been in the realm of student and resident education.

Scan the QR code below or enter the YouTube link to watch the entire interview with Dr. D. Craig Miller conducted by Walter J. McCarthy, MD, brought to you by the SVS History Project Work Group.

 http://tinyurl.com/MillerXDC

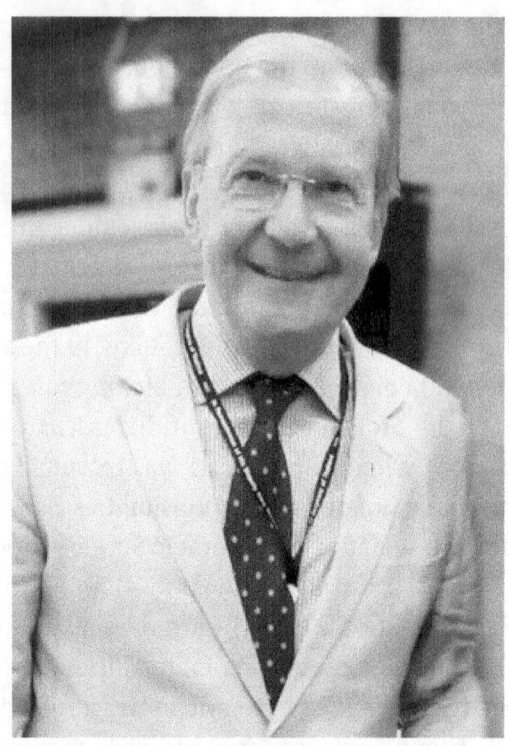

Frans L. Moll, MD

Frans Moll was born in the Netherlands in 1950. His father was an engineer involved in ship building in Delft. His uncle and grandfather were both physicians. He entered medicine with a focus on gynecology-obstetrics but was persuaded to choose vascular surgery by Professor Theo Theodorides in Utrecht. Frans met his wife-to-be, a surgical OR nurse, during his residency at St. Antonius Hospital in Utrecht, and together they have had three children.

After his general surgical training in the Netherlands, Dr. Moll spent significant time in the United States. For one year he did post-doctoral research in vascular surgery at UCLA under Dr. Wesley Moore. After that he moved for a second year of training to Seattle, learning duplex applications for peripheral artery disease with Dr. Eugene Strandness in 1980. When Dr. Moll returned to the Netherlands, Dr. Strandness asked two of the Seattle bloodflow technologists to travel to Utrecht for six months to introduce duplex ultrasound techniques in the Netherlands.

Dr. Moll is well-known for developing the Moll Ring Cutter, used in remote endarterectomy of the superficial femoral artery. This came to market with the assistance of the Fogarty Institute in California. His device simplifies a closed superficial femoral endarterectomy, allowing the operation to be done with only one incision instead of two. Dr. Moll also conceived of a percutaneous implantable biological venous valve, which he brought to clinical trials but was never marketed.

Dr. Moll served as Chairman of the Board for Vascular Education of the Dutch Society for Vascular Surgery from 2005–2012. Dr. Moll also has been a program co-chairman for the annual Charing Cross Symposium in London since 2009. In addition, he has served as a scientific committee and faculty member for the annual Veith Symposium in New York since 1996. Dr. Moll has been Professor of Surgery and Head of the Department of Surgery of the University Medical Center in Utrecht, utilizing his philosophy of building an excellent team of surgeons using empathy rather than the old traditional European autocratic method. He reserves one-and-a-half days per week to operate. He focuses on open thoraco-abdominal aneurysm repair, re-do aortic and re-do carotid surgery and is a specialist in resecting glomus tumors of the carotid region.

Scan the QR code below or enter the YouTube link to watch the entire interview with Dr. Frans L. Moll conducted by Kenneth J. Cherry, MD, and James S.T. Yao, MD, brought to you by the SVS History Project Work Group.

 http://tinyurl.com/MollXF2

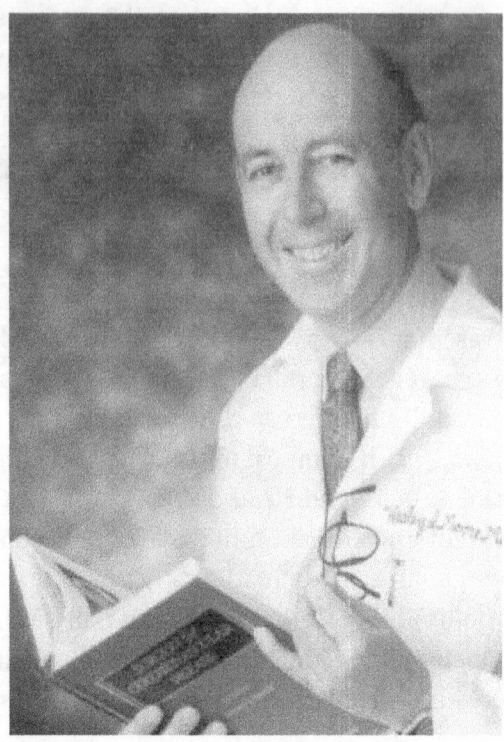

Wesley S. Moore, MD

Wesley Moore was born in San Bernardino, California in 1935. The youngest of three children, Wes suffered from severe childhood asthma that was affected by the climate and air quality of his home town. Consequently, in 1944 his family moved to Palm Springs, California. Also because of his asthma, Wes was home-schooled until ninth grade. He recalls that both of his parents were immigrants and neither was highly proficient in English, however, his father was extremely good at mathematics.

Wes chose the University of California San Francisco (USCF) for college and graduated with a major in biochemistry. He was accepted into the medical school there, graduating in 1959. He remembers always knowing that he wanted to become a physician because, with his asthma, he had had so much contact with doctors and admired them.

Dr. Moore completed his internship and surgical residency at UCSF, where he was greatly inspired by F. William Blaisdell, who was at that time the chief of surgery at the San Francisco VA Hospital. Dr. Moore recalls being scrubbed on the famous, world's first-ever axillary to femoral artery bypass, which was performed at the San Francisco VA in 1962. Dr. Moore was the second-year resident taking care of a patient who required an aorto-bi-femoral bypass. The patient had a pre-existing above-knee amputation on one side, and the team completed the operation with an aortic to femoral artery bypass on the other side. The following day the bypass graft thrombosed, resulting in severe ischemia from the mid-abdomen distally. The team returned the patient to the operating room immediately where the patient had a cardiac arrest but was resuscitated with external chest compression. Faced with this difficult circumstance, Dr. Blaisdell envisioned an axillary to femoral artery bypass, which would restore circulation without requiring the abdomen to be re-opened. The surgical team cut down on the axillary artery and re-opened the groin incision. They then performed a lateral tunnel with an external vein stripper instrument through which they could pull the bypass graft. Dr. Moore recalls that the patient did fairly well and survived for five more years. This and other interesting events during his residency convinced Dr. Moore that he wanted to be a vascular surgeon.

Following surgical residency, Dr. Moore was drafted into the Army and became a Captain. He soon became Chief of Surgery of the 98th General Hospital in Munich, Germany. Soon after his military experience, he spent 1967 to 1968 studying carotid artery disease as a NIH research fellow.

Dr. Moore's first surgical faculty position was when he returned to UCSF, but he was soon recruited to become the Chief of Vascular Surgery at the University of Arizona in Tucson. In 1980, the pioneering vascular surgeon Wylie Barker retired as the chief of vascular surgery at UCLA. Wesley Moore was the obvious choice for the position, and many of Dr. Moore's most important accomplishments and contributions followed at UCLA.

With his long interest in the surgical treatment of the carotid artery, and also his basic science background, Dr. Moore became a very important participant and intellectual leader in the multiple randomized controlled studies of this disease. He also published an early definitive carotid textbook and numerous book chapters to help other surgeons understand the concepts.

Dr. Moore was a surgeon who early on appreciated the potential of endovascular treatment for aortic aneurysms. He contributed much to this field and is in fact credited with having invented the term "endovascular surgery." The first commercially manufactured aortic stent graft was produced by a company called Endovascular Technology or EVT. When it came time to place the first-ever EVT graft in a human, Dr. Moore was chosen to be the surgeon. The procedure was completed successfully on February 10, 1993. The first graft he implanted was a tube graft, but by September 1994, Dr. Moore was using EVT bifurcated grafts as well.

Beginning in 1982, the American Board of Surgery offered a certificate of "Special Qualification in Vascular Surgery" based on passing a challenging examination. Dr. Moore realized that a well-designed vascular surgery review course would be useful. He has ever since directed this course, often with the help of others at UCLA. His review course has been attended by most vascular surgeons and most vascular surgery fellows for nearly 40 years. The course is accompanied by a textbook called *Vascular and Endovascular Surgery: A Comprehensive Review*. This outstanding and invaluable text has been kept up-to-date with multiple editions.

In addition to his many other contributions, Dr. Moore has maintained a busy, comprehensive vascular surgery practice and mentored numerous surgical trainees and vascular fellows. For all of these accomplishments, he has received many honors, including being elected the president of the Society for Vascular Surgery in 1985 and, in 2011, being awarded a lifetime achievement award by the SVS.

Dr. Moore is an avid tennis player and enjoys skiing and traveling with his family. He is happily married and has two sons, Edward and Michael.

Scan the QR code below or enter the YouTube link to watch the entire interview with Dr. Wesley S. Moore conducted by Roger T. Gregory, MD, brought to you by the SVS History Project Work Group.

 http://tinyurl.com/MooreXW1

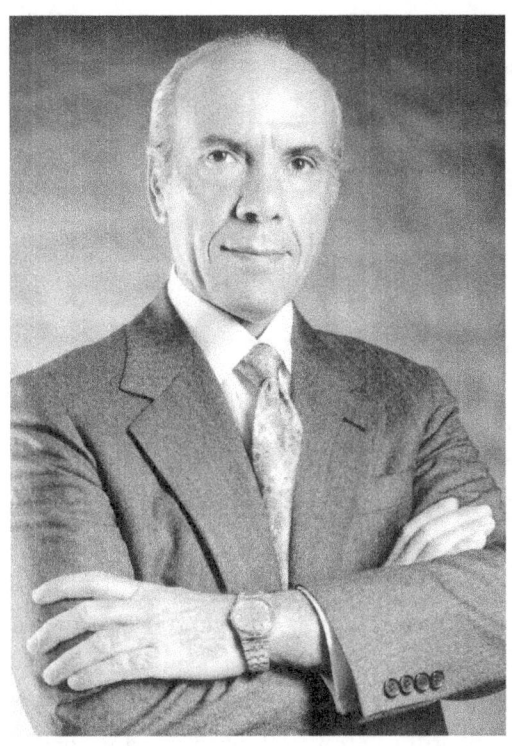

Hassan Najafi, MD

Hassan Najafi's life story is a remarkable sequence of events that carried him from his birth in Tehran, Iran on May 22, 1930 to world renown as a surgical leader in the United States. He ultimately became Chair of the Department of Cardiovascular and Thoracic Surgery at Rush Presbyterian-St. Luke's Medical Center, now Rush University Medical Center, in 1972 at age 42. He held that leadership position, directing cardiac, vascular and thoracic surgery for 25 years. Through that role, he became a national and international figure in cardiothoracic surgery and also in vascular surgery.

Growing up in Tehran, Hassan was an excellent student. He recalls that his father, who was a dairy farmer with no formal education, had two instructions for him. He should become a physician, and he should marry a westerner. Najafi was admitted to medical school at the University of Tehran where he graduated first in his class of 242 students in 1954. While in high school, he had become an excellent table tennis player, and eventually became captain of the national Iranian team. Because of his skill, while he was still in medical school, he was invited to meet and play table tennis with the Shah of Iran and the Shah's wife, Queen Soraya. These games occurred weekly for many months!

After one year of internship and two years of surgical training in Iran, he received a government scholarship to support two years of study abroad. He chose the United States, likely inspired by reading about John H. Gibbon's famous first use of cardiopulmonary bypass to repair an atrial septal defect on May 6, 1953. When Dr. Najafi arrived in the United States, the first thing he did was travel by bus to Philadelphia to meet with Dr. Gibbon. Dr. Najafi eventually obtained an internship in Washington, DC and the following year began general surgery training at St. Luke's Hospital in Chicago. During his training, he was greatly influenced by the pioneer cardiac and vascular surgeons Ormond Julian, Samuel Dye and Hushang Javid.

After training, Dr. Najafi joined this renowned group at Rush Presbyterian-St. Luke's Hospital. There followed a legendary clinical practice, which included all types of complex cardiac and vascular surgery. Of note, Dr. Najafi performed the first heart transplant in Chicago in 1968. Additionally, he had a special interest and skill related to thoracic aorta, aortic arch, aortic dissection, and thoracoabdomial aneurysm surgery. He took great pride in eventually having trained over 56 surgeons in these areas.

Dr. Najafi's many honors and leadership positions include being the first president of the Thoracic Surgery Directors Association in 1975 and serving as Chairman of the American Board of Thoracic Surgery from 1985 to 1987. He also served as President of the Society for Thoracic Surgery from 1982 until 1983.

Related to vascular surgery, Dr. Najafi served as a member of the Vascular Surgery Training Subcommittee of the Residency Review Committee for Surgery from 1976 to 1978. He was an important part of the initiative recommending that the American Board of Medical Specialties and the American Board of Surgery grant a separate certification in vascular surgery. He was program director of an ACGME vascular surgery fellowship, which he established at Rush University in 1987 and headed until his retirement in 1997. During the 1980s, he participated with the American Board of Surgery in administering oral examinations for vascular surgery.

Hassan Najafi married Marsha Dunn in 1959, and together they raised four children. It is said that he valued the importance of family togetherness above all else. When Dr. Najafi died on May 22, 2017, those who knew him well had lost someone very special. He was a surgeon with superb technical skills, encompassing cardiac and major aortic surgery in a way that few others could match. He was a person of elegance in his appearance and style, yet with humility in his demeanor. He was a master conversationalist, storyteller and public speaker and also an eloquent writer. He was always dedicated to his patients, family and colleagues beyond words, a very exceptional person.

Scan the QR code below or enter the YouTube link to watch the entire interview with Dr. Hassan Najafi conducted by William H. Baker, MD, and James S.T. Yao, MD, brought to you by the SVS History Project Work Group.

 http://tinyurl.com/NajafiXH

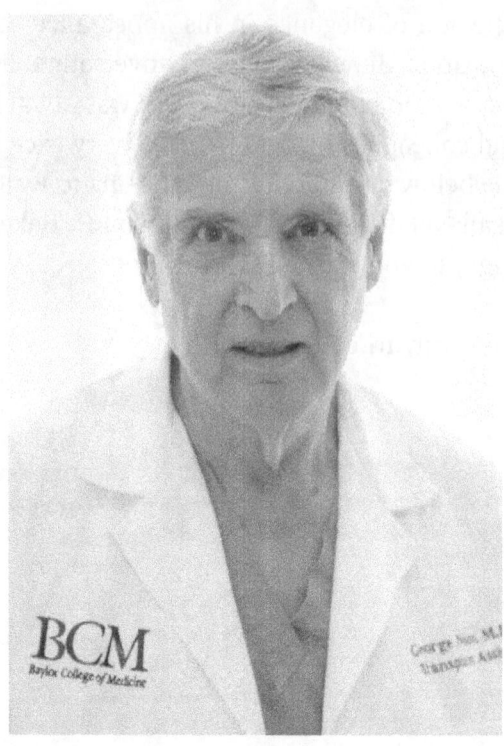

George P. Noon, MD

George Noon was born in Arizona, the son of a nurse mother and a surgeon father. After going to Houston, Texas to the Baylor College of Medicine (1960), he stayed there for his entire career. He went to Baylor after he heard of Michael DeBakey. Noon became his student, then his trusted colleague in surgery, and finally, Dr. DeBakey's surgeon when the great man needed his ascending aorta replaced at age 97.

Dr. Noon practiced general surgery, vascular surgery, cardiac surgery, heart-transplant surgery and cardiac device placement until the day he retired. Michael DeBakey said if he himself ever needed surgery, George Noon should be the one to do it, and as noted, this came to pass.

Dr. Noon became a professor of surgery at a very young age and eventually amassed more than 350 publications. He was a superb clinical surgeon and attributed this to his truly massive experience in the early days of vascular and cardiac surgery. Dr. Noon was the Meyer-DeBakey Professor of Investigative Surgery at the Baylor College of Medicine. During his career, besides his monumental clinical work and teaching of students and clinical trainees, his research focused on organ transplantation and cardiac-assist devices. In 1968, Dr. Noon did the background surgical research that allowed him and Dr. DeBakey to perform their first heart transplant and also their first heart-lung transplants. These were among the first such operations in the United States.

In November 1996, Dr. Noon traveled with Dr. DeBakey to Moscow to consult on the coronary bypass operation planned for the Russian President, Boris Yeltsin. Mr. Yeltsin's Russian cardiac surgeon, Renat S. Akchurin, had previously been one of their trainees in Houston. The operation went well. Dr. Noon was quoted from Moscow by the *New York Times* as saying, "Dr. Akchurin did a very nice operation on the President."

During his remarkable time in practice, Dr. Noon received many honors including the Michael Debakey Humanitarian Award in 2009. One of the most interesting honors he received was related to his working with NASA to develop an axial blood flow pump. This resulted in Dr. Noon being inducted into the Space Technology Hall of Fame.

Scan the QR code below or enter the YouTube link to watch the entire interview with Dr. George P. Noon conducted by Roger T. Gregory, MD, and James S.T. Yao, MD, brought to you by the SVS History Project Work Group.

 http://tinyurl.com/NoonXG1

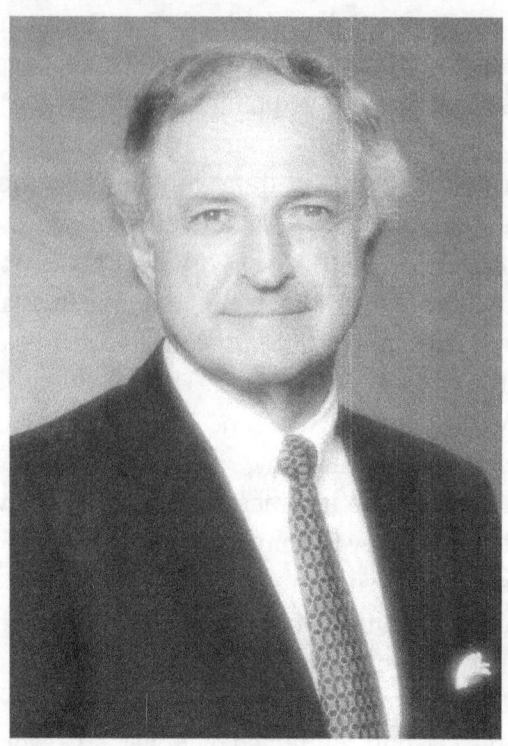

John L. Ochsner, MD

John Ochsner was born in Madison, Wisconsin in 1927. At that time, his father, Alton, was a surgical faculty member at the University of Wisconsin, but he was recruited to Tulane in New Orleans when John was only three months old. John's childhood in New Orleans juxtaposed him among many of the leading vascular surgeons in the United States. That he eventually went on to have a truly remarkable career in both cardiac and vascular surgery himself is not surprising.

John's father had been recruited to Tulane to become the chief of surgery at the time when Rudolph Matas retired. Dr. Matas is considered by many to be the father of vascular surgery in the United States and became a close family friend of the Ochsners. Young John had many memories of visiting the Matas home during childhood. Later, during medical school at Tulane, John and other medical students read medical articles aloud to Dr. Matas, who in old age was nearly blind.

John's father had a considerable interest in vascular surgery and was a founding member of the Society for Vascular Surgery and notably served as its first president when the group met at the Dennis Hotel in Atlantic City, New Jersey on June 8, 1947.

Another remarkable coincidence involves Michael DeBakey, who was a prominent medical student at Tulane when John was a young child. John's father, as Surgical Chairman, was mentoring and advising young DeBakey. DeBakey sometimes would babysit for the Ochsners' children. Thus, John knew Dr. DeBakey well when he arrived in Houston for much of his surgical training years later.

John traveled to the Darlington School, a boarding school in Rome, Georgia for high school. When he graduated, World War II was raging, but being only 17, he was too young to enlist in the army. Therefore, he found a position in the United States Merchant Marine Academy at Kingspoint, New York and trained to be a merchant marine sailor. He spent the remainder of World War II traversing the North Atlantic transporting war material on freighters.

John then went to college and medical school at Tulane and completed a surgical internship at the University of Michigan. In Ann Arbor he met his wife, Mary Lou, to whom he was married until the day he died on July 6, 2018 at the age of 91. Together they had four children.

After internship, he was drafted through the doctors' draft during the Korean War. When he returned from the military, he headed to Houston for his surgical training under Dr. DeBakey. At the Texas Medical Center, he was trained by such notable surgeons as Paul Jordan, Stanley Crawford, Denton Cooley and, of course, Michael DeBakey.

Although he was offered a position on the staff after training with Dr. DeBakey, the young Dr. Ochsner decided to practice at the Ochsner Clinic. This organization, the largest medical clinic in the southern United States, had been founded by his father and several other physicians in 1942. John Ochsner became the chief of surgery at the clinic in 1966 and practiced cardiac and vascular surgery there for 57 years. He oversaw the groundbreaking development of the clinic from the standpoint of research, teaching and clinical care and personally performed more than 12,000 operations.

During Dr. Ochsner's career he held many important national leadership roles and was the president of ten surgical societies. These included many of the most important thoracic surgical societies and also the International Society for Cardiovascular Surgery. Dr. Ochsner played an important role in bringing the *Journal of Vascular Surgery* to life in 1984. He was appointed the chairman of the committee to organize the *Journal*. His committee included

Emerick Szilagyi, Ronald Baird and Calvin Ernst. The original idea for the *Journal* was Dr. DeBakey's, thus the committee assigned him to be the first editor. This seemed appropriate considering that he was "the father of modern vascular surgery" and had had the idea!

Dr. Ochsner had worked with Mosby, the well-known medical publishing company, related to his experience in the thoracic surgery societies, and he therefore recommended that Mosby become the *Journal*'s publisher. This fortuitous arrangement allowed the Society for Vascular Surgery to hold the copyright of the *Journal*, and also allowed the Society to sustain a significant annual profit from its publication.

Throughout his long life, besides his many other honors, John Ochsner was crowned the Rex of Mardi Gras in 1990. This allowed him to follow in his father's footsteps, as Alton had held that same position in 1948.

Scan the QR code below or enter the YouTube link to watch the entire interview with Dr. John L. Ochsner conducted by Roger T. Gregory, MD, brought to you by the SVS History Project Work Group.

 Interview 1: http://tinyurl.com/OchXJ1

 Interview 2: http://tinyurl.com/OchXJ2

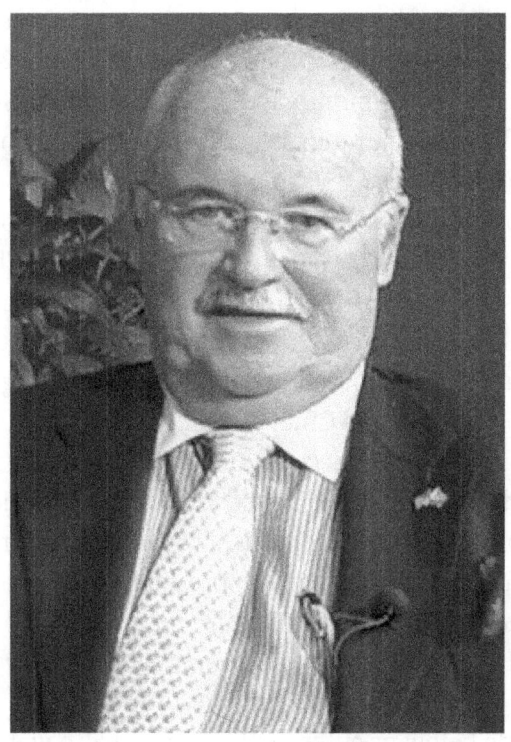

Thomas F. O'Donnell, Jr., MD

Thomas O'Donnell was born in Providence, Rhode Island on September 7, 1941. His father was a high school principal. Tom attended St. Sebastian's prep school in Newton, Massachusetts and had a football injury in high school, a femur fracture, that introduced him to medical care. He was so impressed by his treatment that he decided to become a surgeon. Tom was soon afterwards admitted to Harvard College where he majored in Classics, Latin and Greek and served as an editor of the *Harvard Crimson*, the college daily newspaper.

Tom attended Tufts University Medical School from 1963 through 1967, rotating on the surgery service at the Boston City Hospital, which is where he eventually ended up completing his general surgery training.

During his surgical training, due to the Vietnam War Berry draft plan, he spent two years in the Marine Corps serving at the Parris Island base in South Carolina.

Returning to Boston to complete his surgical residency, Dr. O'Donnell continued to work with an important surgical mentor, George H.A. Clowes. Dr. Clowes helped to arrange a special fellowship at St. Thomas' Hospital in London with professors John Kinmonth and Norman Browse. His year in London, 1974–75, initiated his lifelong interest in lymphatic and venous research and the related clinical treatment.

Returning to Boston, Dr. O'Donnell completed a formal, one-year vascular fellowship at the Massachusetts General Hospital under R. Clement Darling, Jr.

After his fellowship, he returned to his medical school alma mater, Tufts, as a young vascular surgeon which allowed him to work with two distinguished senior vascular surgeons, Allan Callow and Ralph Deterling. In the years that followed Dr. O'Donnell became Chief of Vascular Surgery and then the Chairman of the Department of Surgery at Tufts. He was eventually asked to become the CEO and President of the Tufts-New England Medical Center. In that role he learned to become an accomplished medical administrator. His leadership skills also led him to become the president of many surgical societies including the American Venous Forum in 1998 and the Society for Vascular Surgery in 2001. Dr. O'Donnell has authored more than 275 papers and textbook chapters.

Scan the QR code below or enter the YouTube link to watch the entire interview with Dr. Thomas F. O'Donnell, Jr., conducted by William H. Baker, MD, and James S.T. Yao, MD, brought to you by the SVS History Project Work Group.

 http://tinyurl.com/ODonXT

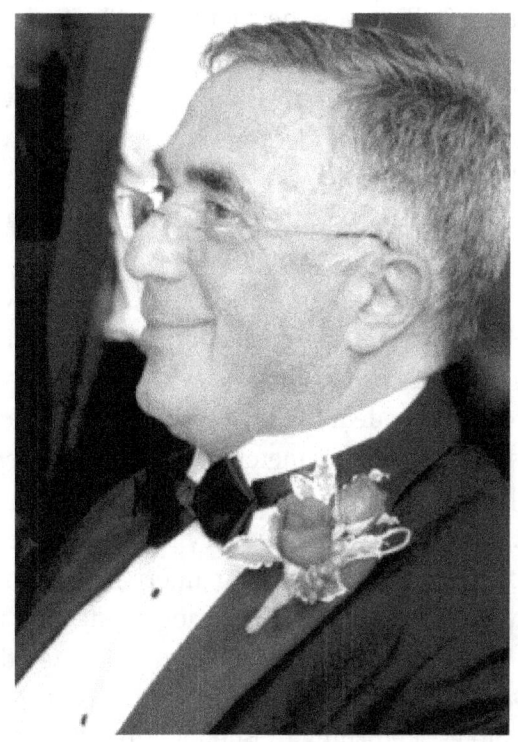

Juan Carlos Parodi, MD

Juan Parodi was born in Buenos Aires, Argentina in 1942. His father was a businessman, and his mother was a teacher. There were four children in the family; three became engineers, but Juan was inspired by two teachers to a lifelong interest in biology. These two high school "professors" taught anatomy and biology and were also both surgeons. His school was in a suburb of Buenos Aires where many British railroad company executives lived, and the classes were taught in English. Juan began his medical studies in his home town of Buenos Aires where college was combined with medical school. He received his MD from the Universidad del Salvador in Buenos Aires in 1968. He continued to pursue general surgical training, also in Buenos Aires, finishing in 1972.

Dr. Parodi continued his education by accepting post-graduate surgical fellowships first at the University of Illinois in Chicago and then in vascular surgery, in 1975–76, at the Cleveland Clinic. It was as a fellow at the Cleveland Clinic in 1976 that Dr. Parodi conceived the idea for which he became world-famous. During the middle 1970s the Cleveland Clinic was a major referral center for open abdominal aneurysm surgery. As a trainee, Dr Parodi was able to scrub on many such cases with the Clinic's two pioneer vascular surgeons, Al Humphries and Edwin Beven. Despite the extensive experience and tremendous effort of these surgeons, Dr. Parodi observed that some of the frail patients were not able to recover after their open aneurysm surgery. He concluded that a simpler, less-invasive method was needed.

There followed a series of experiments at the Cleveland Clinic during 1976 using a dog model. Dr. Parodi fashioned a homemade small-diameter graft of nylon fabric, also using elastic stainless-steel wire. In a collapsed form this could be introduced retrograde into the dog's aorta for deployment. He found that the device was too large in diameter to pass from the femoral arteries, so he introduced it through the iliac arteries. In 1976, Dr. Parodi and his wife returned home to Argentina for him to begin clinical practice as a vascular surgeon. He continued to pursue his idea of an internal aortic graft. An important advance for Dr. Parodi came in 1988 when, by chance, he met Julio Palmaz for the first time at a meeting in Washington, DC. They discussed the aortic project, and Dr. Palmaz gave him several of his new balloon-expandable metal stents as samples. Returning to Buenos Aires, Dr. Parodi found a manufacturer who could produce the stents in significantly larger diameters that were suitable for aortic applications. He also developed a dog model, where as a first step, a Dacron graft with a central expanded area, "an aneurysm," was first sewn in surgically. At a later date the homemade stent-graft could then be placed for an "aneurysm repair."

By 1990, 42 successful dog operations had been performed. Dr. Parodi then received a phone call from Carlos Menem, president of Argentina at the time. The president had a favor to ask. He had a relative, a man with severe COPD, who had a symptomatic aortic aneurysm. Could Dr. Parodi please take a look at the case?

This phone call led to the world's first successful endovascular abdominal aortic aneurysm repair which took place on September 7, 1990 in Buenos Aires. Dr. Parodi's brilliant idea expanded and evolved, at first through his untiring promotion and enthusiasm, but soon through ingenious modifications by many others. He himself performed, or supervised others who performed, the first demonstration cases in Europe (October 1992) and in the United States (November 23, 1992) and published the first definitive paper of his own first cases in the *Annals of Vascular Surgery* in 1991. After that, inventors, entrepreneurs and industrial engineers have refined the basic concept to the point where the majority of abdominal aortic aneurysms are now repaired worldwide with an endovascular device.

Dr. Parodi never was able to effectively patent his magnificent idea or to achieve significant financial gain from it. However, he has been greatly rewarded and acknowledged in other ways and has undoubtedly become the most famous and honored vascular surgeon in the world over the last 30 years. Among his many honors are the Jacobson Innovation Award from the American College of Surgeons in 2002, the very first Medal for Innovation from the Society for Vascular Surgery in 2006 and also a Lifetime Achievement Award from the Society for Vascular Surgery in 2020.

Another recognition was very special. In 1980, soon after he returned to Argentina from the Cleveland Clinic, Dr. Parodi saved the life of a young priest by removing his gangrenous gallbladder. Dr. Parodi and his wife were recently invited to reunite and spend time with his former patient at the Vatican. The man whose life he had saved was named Jorge Bergoglio, now better known as Pope Francis.

It is of great interest to note that, like many other great inventions, there were other centers in the world working on the same idea. Unknown to Dr. Parodi, a Poland-born Ukrainian cardiovascular surgeon named Nokolai Volodos and his team did extensive work in this area during the 1980s and '90s in the Soviet Union. They successfully repaired a thoracic aortic aneurysm with a trans-femoral access stent graft in 1987. This would be the world's first reported case. They attempted repair of an infra-renal aortic aneurysm in 1989, but a limb became kinked and they had to open the abdomen. It was not until 1993 that they were successful with an abdominal aneurysm. Dr. Volodos' accomplishments were not published in the English literature and were not known in the West at the time.

Scan the QR code below or enter the YouTube link to watch the entire interview with Dr. Juan Carlos Parodi conducted by Melina R. Kibbe, MD, brought to you by the SVS History Project Work Group.

 http://tinyurl.com/ParodiXJC

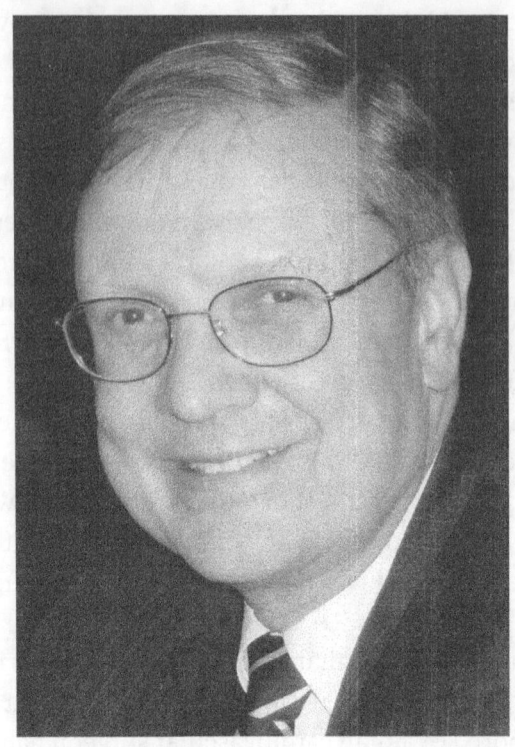

William H. Pearce, MD

Bill Pearce grew up in Colorado Springs, Colorado. He had been born in Pueblo, which is 45 miles south of Colorado Springs, on February 19, 1949. His family's home was on the lower slope of Cheyenne Mountain, very close to where the Broadmoor Hotel is located. Bill's father worked for the National Cash Register Corporation and also did construction work building houses. At an early age Bill was taught many building skills by his father that he still uses around his home. His mother worked in doctor's offices doing the bookkeeping and billing and working as a receptionist.

In high school, Bill was a very good tennis player and skier, but also an excellent student. He was accepted at many colleges, including Stanford, Yale and Harvard. Harvard won out thanks to the best scholarship possibility. Bill graduated from Harvard cum laude in 1971. His lifetime love of tennis continued to play a role as he taught tennis at hotels and country clubs during summer breaks during college and up through his second year of medical school to help with expenses.

Bill returned to the University of Colorado for medical school and was initially interested in a career in internal medicine. During his second year of medical school Bill married his high school friend, Ann Arnold.

Bill was accepted into a medical internship at the Mayo Clinic in Rochester, Minnesota, but partway through the year decided that surgery was his true calling. He returned to the University of Colorado where he finished as chief surgical resident in 1981. Dr. Pearce was initially very interested in cardiac surgery and also had extensive experience with transplant surgery, given that Thomas Starzl was the chief of surgery at that time. However, Bill remembers operating with his attending, Bob Rutherford, repairing the brachial artery of a young child as the moment when he decided to make vascular surgery his career. Dr. Rutherford, Bill's lifelong mentor, contacted several vascular surgery program directors, and Bill ended up traveling for a vascular fellowship to Northwestern in Chicago. He names his teachers there, James Yao and John Bergan, as his other career mentors.

Immediately after finishing the vascular fellowship, Bill and Ann spent two years in Cincinnati working with Dick Kempczinski, and then returned to the University of Colorado for four years.

In 1988, James Yao at Northwestern was able to recruit Bill to return to Chicago. Much of Bill's tremendously productive career was spent at Northwestern. He first served as chief of the adjacent Lakeside VA vascular service and then became the Northwestern vascular division chief (1998–2010). Dr. Pearce had an extremely busy clinical practice and was an early adopter of endovascular techniques. He placed the first endovascular aortic stent graft in the city of Chicago in 1993.

Besides his clinical responsibilities, which included teaching vascular fellows, Dr. Pearce developed a highly productive, federal grant supported, research laboratory focusing on aortic aneurysm structure and their causes. He credits his great success and capacity to publish literally hundreds of important papers in this area with his ability to collaborate with talented basic science researchers. Dr. Pearce's academic contribution also includes co-directing the annual Northwestern December Symposium for many years. Remarkably, Dr. Pearce has produced more than 40 textbooks, including the annual books related to the December Symposium.

Realizing that the U.S. military had very few vascular surgeons, Dr. Pearce was instrumental in establishing the volunteer coverage program for Landstuhl, Germany during the Afghanistan and Iraq wars. This became a successful two-week rotation allowing vascular surgeons to help at the large military hospital at the Landstuhl Air Force Base. Dr. Pearce himself rotated there in 2008 and 2010.

Among his many honors, Dr. Pearce was selected to serve as the president of the American Association for Vascular Surgeons 2001–2002. He has been given numerous faculty teaching awards and humanitarian awards throughout his long career. In 2019, the Society for Vascular Surgery presented Dr. Pearce with its Lifetime Achievement Award for his many contributions. This is the highest honor the Society can bestow on one of its members.

Dr. Pearce and Ann have recently retired to their hometown of Colorado Springs where Bill continues to ski and is often visited by their four children.

Scan the QR code below or enter the YouTube link to watch the entire interview with Dr. William H. Pearce conducted by Roger T. Gregory, MD, brought to you by the SVS History Project Work Group.

 http://tinyurl.com/PearceXW

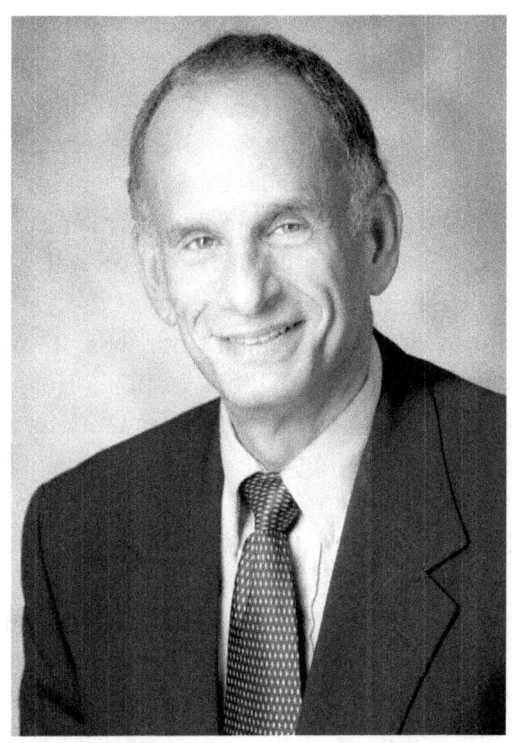

Bruce A. Perler, MD

Bruce Perler grew up in New Bedford, Massachusetts and graduated from the public high school there. His father was a truck mechanic and driver who instilled in Bruce the lifelong principles of hard work, honesty and loyalty. His mother was a Licensed Practical Nurse. Bruce was born on March 12, 1950 in New Bedford and knew from an early age that he wanted to become a surgeon. Family friends suggested to him that Duke University would be a good place for college, and after a visit to the university with his parents, he agreed.

Bruce received an A.B. in Zoology from Duke in 1972, where he was Phi Beta Kappa. He remained in Durham for his MD from the Duke University School of Medicine. Legendary cardiovascular surgeon David Sabiston was the surgical chairman at Duke when Bruce was a student, and he was very involved with the students. Dr. Sabiston wrote letters of recommendation for students, and Bruce ended up being accepted into the premier general surgery residency at the Massachusetts General Hospital (MGH). Dr. Perler decided to stay at the MGH for a one-year vascular fellowship during 1981 and 1982. He was trained by several pioneering master surgeons, including David Brewster and R. Clement Darling Jr.

In 1982 he was recruited to Johns Hopkins by Dr. George Zuidema, who was the chairman there from 1964 until 1984. Dr. Perler's many career accomplishments and honors have occurred with Hopkins as his base. These include being named the first recipient of the Julius H. Jacobson II, MD Endowed Chair in Vascular Surgery. He has served as Director of the Vascular Noninvasive Laboratory at the Johns Hopkins Hospital since 1982. In 1998, he established a vascular surgery fellowship at the Johns Hopkins Hospital and served as director until 2009. Dr. Perler considers open operations for complex aortic disease among the most interesting cases, with carotid endarterectomy as his favorite. Dr. Perler was named the Chief of the Division of Vascular Surgery & Endovascular Therapy at Johns Hopkins in January, 2002 at the time when Melville Williams retired.

In addition to his busy surgical practice and leadership at Hopkins, Dr. Perler has edited or co-edited five textbooks, including as co-editor with his friend Anton Sidawy of *Rutherford's Textbook of Vascular Surgery and Endovascular Therapy*. He has authored more than 200 medical journal articles and textbook chapters and has served on the editorial boards of four vascular surgery journals. From 2009 to 2016, he served as the Senior Editor of the *Journal of Vascular Surgery (JVS)*, again with Dr. Sidawy. During their time as editors of the *JVS* they established the two sister journals, *Journal of Vascular Surgery: Venous & Lymphatic Disorders* and the *Journal of Vascular Surgery: Cases*.

From 2015–2016, Dr. Perler served as president of the Society for Vascular Surgery and then from 2016–2017 as chair of the SVS Foundation. He had previously served as president of the Southern Association for Vascular Surgery in 2009–2010, the Eastern Vascular Society in 2005–2006 and the Chesapeake Vascular Society. In 2016, Dr. Perler was selected to serve as the Associate Executive Director of the American Board of Surgery for Vascular Surgery when Robert Rhodes retired from that position.

Scan the QR code below or enter the YouTube link to watch the entire interview with Dr. Bruce A. Perler conducted by Walter J. McCarthy, MD, and Richard A. Lynn, MD, brought to you by the SVS History Project Work Group.

 http://tinyurl.com/PerlerXB

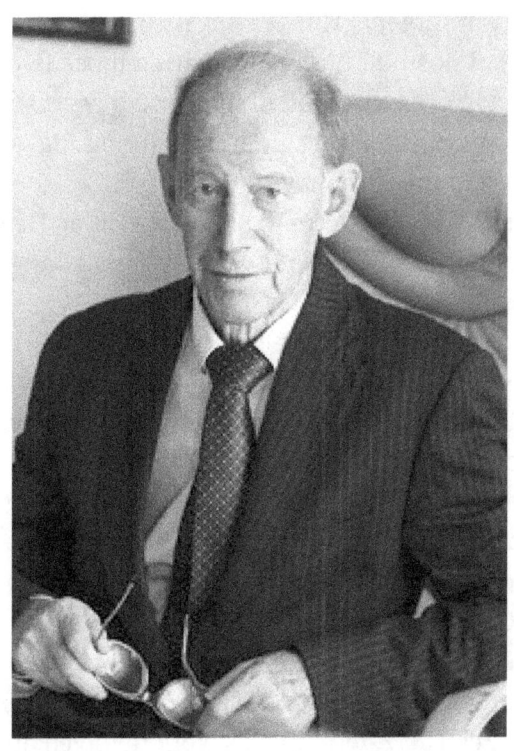

Anatoly V. Pokrovsky, MD

Anatoly Vladimirovich Pokrovsky was born on November 21, 1930 in the city of Minsk, Belarus, which was then part of the Soviet Union. Both of his parents were obstetrician-gynecologists. In 1935, his father accepted a position to be the chair of gynecology at a new university in Khabarovsk, in the far east of Russia. Later the family re-settled in Moscow where Anatoly finished his education and also had his medical training.

In 1959, Anatoly joined the recently founded Institute of Thoracic Surgery under the USSR Academy of Medical Sciences in Moscow. His surgery focused on the new field of cardiac surgery at a time when vascular surgery had not been established as a separate entity. He recalls operations early in his career, before cardio-pulmonary bypass was possible. In these he used his index finger for finger fracture mitral valve commisurotomy to relieve mitral valve stenosis.

As vascular surgery cases became more common, his surgical chairman at the Bakulev Scientific Center for Cardiovascular Surgery in Moscow appointed him chief of vascular surgery. This was in 1966, when he was 36 years old, and he served in that position until 1986. During those two decades, Dr. Pokrovsky also worked in organ transplantation and developed fabric prosthesis for aorta repair. He recalls hand-fashioning a fabric tube graft using material from a lady's blouse in the early days of this work.

In the 1980s, Dr. Pokrovsky accepted the position as Head of the Vascular Surgery Department of the Institute of Surgery named after A.V. Vishnevsky and remained there for the remainder of his career.

In 1986 Dr. Pokrovsky was involved in the creation of the Angiology and Vascular Surgery Society in Russia. In 1994, he established and became editor of the quarterly, bilingual journal, *Angiology and Vascular Surgery*. Several years later in 2000, Dr. Pokrovsky was the first Russian surgeon to be selected to serve as president of the European Society of Vascular Surgery. He had long supported international intellectual exchange in medicine and first traveled to the United States to attend a Society for Vascular Surgery (SVS) meeting in 1973. Dr. Pokrovsky was an honorary member of the SVS.

Dr. Pokrovsky recalled many vascular surgical firsts that have taken place in Russia, going as far back as the 1800s. These include the experimental work in dogs by Nikolai Eck (1847–1908). Eck's work involved an attempt to understand portal vein and liver function by creating side-to-side portal vein to vena caval fistulas. This included ligation of the hepatic portal vein in-flow to isolate the liver from portal blood flow. This became the so-called "Eck fistula" that was studied in much more detail by another Russian, Ivan Pavlov, with work that was published in 1893. Pavlov, who was a physiologist, and his co-author surgeons studied 20 dogs, diverting portal vein blood to the vena cava. They demonstrated hepatic encephelopathy, particularly when the dogs were fed a "meat diet." Dr. Pokrovsky also related the experimental use of the first "heart-lung" bypass machine, used in animals in Russia in 1920. He also knew personally the Ukrainian surgeon, Dr. Nicolai Volodos, who is credited with performing the earliest endovascular aortic procedure. This involved placing a homemade stent-graft to repair a post-traumatic thoracic aneurysm in 1987. Dr. Pokrovsky reflects that many surgical techniques and devices that were pioneered in Russia and the Soviet Union were unrecognized worldwide due to a lack of industrial follow-through.

Dr. Pokrovsky himself pioneered many first-time vascular surgery operations in his country. In 1962, he performed the first ascending aortic repair in the USSR and in 1965 resected an aortic dissection of the descending aorta. In 1972, he repaired an aortic arch aneurysm with prosthetic reconstruction of the great vessels. Dr. Pokrovsky is credited with, for the first time in the world in 1971, performing a trans-aortic endarterectomy of the celiac, superior mesenteric and bilateral renal arteries. He was also one of the first surgeons in Russia to perform carotid endarterectomy and notably was an early proponent of the eversion technique for that operation.

It is said that Anatoly Vladimirovich Pokrovsky was the founder of vascular surgery in Russia as we know it today, and that the existence of vascular surgery and angiology as specialties in Russia were his most important accomplishments. Dr. Pokrovsky's advice for young surgeons in his field was, "you must love vascular surgery and work very hard".

Dr. Pokrovsky died on June 2, 2022.

Scan the QR code below or enter the YouTube link to watch the entire interview with Dr. Anatoly V. Pokrovsky conducted by Norman M. Rich, MD, and James S.T. Yao, MD, brought to you by the SVS History Project Work Group.

 http://tinyurl.com/PokrXA

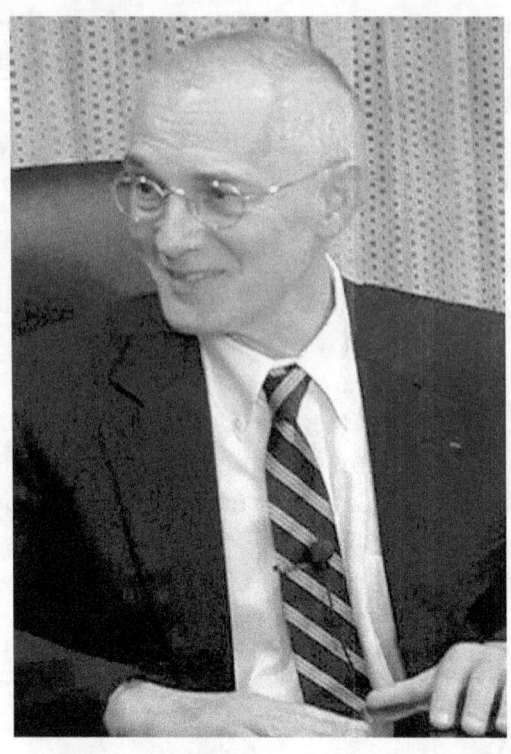

Jean-Baptiste Ricco, MD

Jean Ricco was born in March 1948, in Saint Mandé, France, and he spent his childhood in that suburb of Paris. He studied at the University of Paris La Sorbonne, and then at the Faculty of Medicine René Descartes and Pierre and Marie Curie in Paris. When he was a surgical resident following medical school, he had the opportunity to spend time on the service of Charles Dubost at the Hôpital Broussais. Years before, in 1951, Dr. Dubost had performed the first-ever direct aortic aneurysm repair with a cadaveric homograft preserved by freezing. Dubost had reported this in the *Archives of Surgery* in 1952. Dr. Ricco credits his aspiration to become a vascular surgeon to Dr. Dubost.

    Dr. Ricco was subsequently a chief resident with Professor Edouard Kieffer and separately with Professor Jean-Michel Cormier, both in Paris. These two pioneering vascular surgeons had quite different styles. Professor Cormier was a more-classical surgeon who came from general surgery and taught Dr.

Ricco much about technical vascular surgery. Dr. Kieffer was very modern in his approach, focusing on the biggest, most technically complicated vascular cases. Dr. Kieffer was also interested in writing about his experience, which was quite unique in France at that time. Dr. Kieffer had cases coming from all over the Mediterranean area to his clinic.

Following general surgery training, Dr. Ricco received a research grant from the Fulbright Foundation and used that to travel to Northwestern University in Chicago for a two-year vascular fellowship under doctors John J. Bergan and James S.T. Yao between 1982 and 1983. During his time in Chicago, doctors William Pearce and Linda Graham were the other vascular fellows, and Walter McCarthy was the chief resident on the service.

Returning to France, Dr. Ricco earned a PhD in biostatistics and epidemiology in 1985. He was soon named Professor of Vascular Surgery at the University of Poitiers in 1990 and began leadership of the Department of Vascular Surgery that year. At Poitiers, he developed a busy clinical career and was particularly interested in carotid surgery, aneurysms, thoracoabdominal aneurysms, and lower extremity bypass. In addition, his dedication to clinical research and publication led to his appointment as the editor-in-chief of the *European Journal of Vascular Surgery* in 2010. He has served as president of the French Society for Vascular Surgery from 2009 to 2010 and was elected as president of the European Society for Vascular Surgery in 2014. In 2003, Dr. Ricco became a member and Distinguished Fellow of the Society for Vascular Surgery.

Dr. Ricco has a deeply held belief in applying his medical skills in humanitarian causes, particularly in Southeast Asia. He established an institute at the University of Ho Chi Minh City to develop academic vascular and endovascular surgery and to teach those techniques. Besides teaching and operating in Vietnam, he also routinely accepts Vietnamese surgical trainees at his own institution in France. For these efforts, he was honored by the president of France, Jacques Chirac, with the Chevalier de la Legion d'Honneur in 2000. Dr. Ricco explains the background of that unique, high honor as being related to an encounter with the French president in Cambodia. Dr. Ricco and his medical team were working in rural Cambodia at the time. Along with other projects, they were helping to prepare walking prostheses for children who had required amputation after encountering leftover anti-personnel landmines from the time of the Khmer Rouge onslaught. One day, President Chirac, who happened to be touring Cambodia, came unannounced to their facility by helicopter. The President was very interested in what they were doing, and he spent an hour touring their facility and had coffee with the group. When he left, he told Dr. Ricco, "I will remember you and your team." About six weeks later, Dr. Ricco received a call from the President's office and soon after was awarded the Legion of Honor.

Dr. Ricco and his wife have three adult children, all whom live and work in different countries around the world.

Scan the QR code below or enter the YouTube link to watch the entire interview with Dr. Jean-Baptiste Ricco conducted by Walter J. McCarthy, MD, and James S.T. Yao, MD, brought to you by the SVS History Project Work Group.

 http://tinyurl.com/RiccoXJB

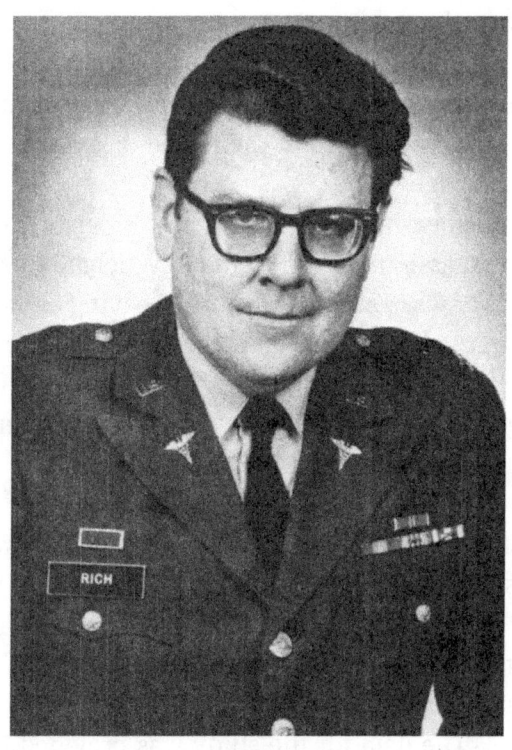

Norman M. Rich, MD

Norman Minner Rich was born in Ray, Arizona in 1934. Now a ghost town, at the time of his birth the community served a large copper mine of the same name. Almost everyone in the town worked in the mines, but both of Norman's parents taught school. It was their dedication to higher education, Norman says, that led him to pursue college instead of taking a job in the mines. He was drawn toward a career in medicine by the family's physician, who had been a World War I military surgeon and shared his stories and textbooks with him. He was also intrigued to learn the principles of trauma first aid in the Boy Scouts.

Norman received a "full ride" scholarship to the University of Arizona, but after two years, he transferred to Stanford; his father and family physician had both attended Stanford, and they encouraged the transfer. He finished his undergraduate degree at Stanford in 1956, where he remained for medical school and graduated in 1960.

Norman was advised to get his military draft obligation taken care of early, so he arranged for an internship at Tripler Army Hospital in Honolulu. Following that year, he began general surgery residency training at Letterman Army General Hospital, which was then at the Presidio of San Francisco, just east of the Golden Gate Bridge.

When Dr. Rich finished his general surgery residency, he went almost immediately to a combat assignment in Vietnam. When he was there in 1965 and 1966, the Vietnam War was gaining full stride. Leaving his wife and three children behind, he departed with his medical group by ship from San Diego for a 30-day trip across the Pacific. Dr. Rich was assigned to be the chief of surgery at the second surgical hospital in An Khe, which is in the central highlands of Vietnam. Ground combat was occurring all around the hospital. It was also the home base to the First Air Cavalry Division with more than 500 helicopters, some of which were used for casualty evacuation to An Khe.

Fortunately fresh from his general surgery training, Dr. Rich recalls virtually 24/7 surgical activity, involving all types of general, neurological, urologic and vascular surgery. During this time, he developed what has become known as the Vietnam vascular registry, in which he kept track of vascular surgical procedures. The data for the study was provided by more than 600 young surgeons who served in Vietnam over the following eight-year period. Dr. Rich reflects that one motivation to do this came from a Marine Corps general who told him, "make something good out of this horrible mess." The registry project led to the publication of a textbook entitled *Vascular Trauma*, which was written with Frank Spencer, who included experience from the Korean War. The registry database, the subsequent organization of blood vessel trauma, and the textbook publication truly represent one of Dr. Rich's most important legacies. The textbook, as of 2022 called *Rich's Vascular Trauma*, is in its fourth edition; it now also includes military data from Afghanistan and the Gulf Wars, as well as from civilian trauma. Control of the publication is now maintained by the Society for Vascular Surgery.

When he returned from Vietnam, Dr. Rich became the first vascular fellow at Walter Reed Hospital in Washington, DC. Soon afterward, he was assigned to be the first chief of vascular surgery at Walter Reed. When the Uniformed Services University of the Health Sciences was established as a federal medical school in 1972, Dr. Rich was named as the first chief of surgery. He was the only full-time surgeon on staff for the school's first five years. In developing the surgical program, he recalls the great organization assistance given to him by such national leaders as David Sabiston from Duke and Michael DeBakey in Houston. He was able to recruit notable surgeons to his staff, including vascular surgeons Harris Schumaker, Charles Rob and Leonel Villavicencio.

Dr. Rich is a member of many professional societies and has been president of six. His military awards include the Legion of Merit, the Bronze Star, the Meritorious Service Award and the Medal of Honor from France (1991). He received the René Leriche Prize from the International Society of Surgery in 2003 and the Michael DeBakey Award from the DeBakey International Surgical Society in 2013. In honor of his many contributions to the field, he also received the Lifetime Achievement Award from the Society for Vascular Surgery.

Dr. Rich has a lifelong passionate interest in surgical and military history and recently has contributed greatly to the Society for Vascular Surgery's History Project Work Group. He credits his professional success to his many mentors and his happy marriage for over 50 years. In 2018, Dr. Rich retired from military service.

Scan the QR code below or enter the YouTube link to watch the entire interview with Dr. Norman M. Rich conducted by Roger T. Gregory, MD, brought to you by the SVS History Project Work Group.

 http://tinyurl.com/RichXN

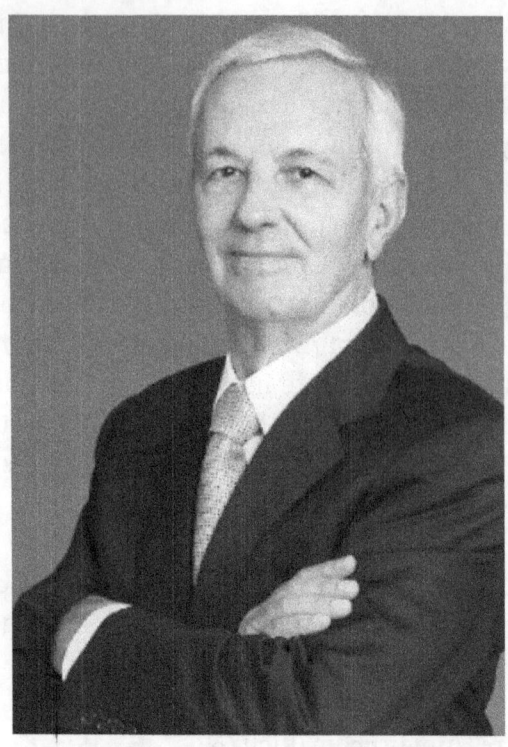

Thomas S. Riles, MD

Thomas Riles was born in 1943 in St. Joseph, Missouri. His father was a general surgeon and his mother a teacher. The family moved to Fort Lauderdale, Florida when Tom was eight, and he completed high school there. His father introduced him to the operating room when he was 13 years old.

Tom attended Stanford University thanks to a generous scholarship. This was followed by medical school at Baylor in Houston, Texas. He completed a year of internship at Baylor and was married that year. As part of the Berry Plan during the Vietnam War, he served as the physician, the diving officer and the radiation officer on a nuclear submarine.

Dr. Riles completed general surgery training from 1972 to 1976 at New York University (NYU) where he was taught by Tony Imparato and Frank Spencer, who he considers lifelong mentors. He became interested in vascular surgery because of the surgical ability to reconstruct diseased arteries.

Dr. Riles joined the NYU faculty and became Chief of Vascular Surgery in

1991. He then concurrently served as Chief of Surgery at NYU for five years after Dr. Spencer retired. In that role he became an early proponent of surgical simulation laboratories and developed that facility at NYU.

Along with his accomplished surgical and academic career, Dr. Riles served as President of the American Association for Vascular Surgery (AAVS). He was instrumental in orchestrating the merger of the two North American vascular societies, the AAVS and the Society for Vascular Surgery (SVS), in 2004. He had previously served as the secretary of the North American chapter of the International Society for Cardiovascular Surgery (NA-ISCVS) during the evolving surgical practice years of the 1990s. During that period other specialties, particularly interventional radiology and cardiology, were threatening vascular surgery's referral base as endovascular techniques allowed the treatment of arterial occlusive disease with catheters. This change in technology, among other issues, made the combination of the two societies attractive. A single society better allowed a unified communication of what vascular disease and vascular surgery were to the public and to the government.

The ISCVS was founded in 1950 as the International Society for Angiology by Dr. Henry Haimovici of Montefiore Medical Center in New York City. The first meeting was held in June 1951, and the ISCVS began holding joint meetings with the SVS in 1967. The SVS functioned as the more academic society, with membership limited to several hundred, and the ISCVS was open to practicing vascular and cardiac surgeons with a larger membership. In 2000, the ISCVS president, John Porter, established a committee which recommended a name change to the American Association for Vascular Surgery. This new name more accurately reflected the Society's members and its mission. Several years later, Dr. Riles was president of this newly named society. During his presidency he worked with Jack Cronenwett, who was president of the SVS, to combine the AAVS and the SVS into one society. The joint association has since been called the Society for Vascular Surgery. This unification, which at the time was controversial and required real political skill to achieve, has been tremendously important and successful.

Scan the QR code below or enter the YouTube link to watch the entire interview with Dr. Thomas S. Riles conducted by Roger T. Gregory, MD, brought to you by the SVS History Project Work Group.

 http://tinyurl.com/RilesXT

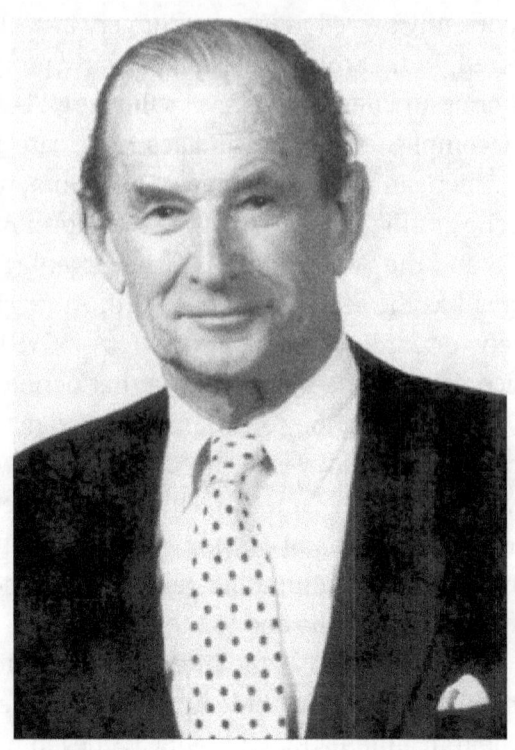

Charles Granville Rob, MD

Charles Rob (May 4, 1913–July 26, 2001) was a pioneer vascular surgeon. After completing his surgical training at St. Thomas' Hospital in London in 1941, he began a long, innovative career that culminated with his position as a professor at the Uniform Services University of Health Sciences in Bethesda, Maryland. Dr. Rob is among the most senior of the interviewed surgeons included in the present series and his experience reflects the early beginnings of vascular arterial surgery right after World War II through the beginning of the endovascular arterial grafting revolution in the 1990s.

Charles was born in Weybridge, England, about 20 miles southwest of central London, where his father practiced medicine as a general practitioner. He often spent time in his father's practice and in high school even assisted with minor surgery, including appendectomies. He followed in his father's footsteps to St. John's College, Cambridge and completed his MD there in 1937. His surgical training followed at St. Thomas' Hospital where he worked continuously throughout the bombardment of London during the Blitz. He recalls the emergency operating rooms being set up in the basement of the hospital and that they conducted elective surgery well outside of London at another hospital in the countryside. Dr. Rob immediately joined the armed forces after completing his surgical training in 1941, joining the airborne paratroopers as a combat surgeon. He was deployed in Tunisia, then in Sicily and on the Italian mainland. At one point he sustained a fractured tibia and patella after a bombing attack. For his service and bravery, he received the Military Cross, which is Great Britain's second highest military award.

Following World War II, Dr. Rob returned to London and at age 37 became the youngest-ever chief of surgery at St. Mary's Hospital. During his years of leadership at St. Mary's, remarkable advances in arterial surgery took place. These included one of the first operations to be performed for symptomatic carotid artery occlusive disease. The 1954 operation, with Dr. Rob's oversight, was accomplished by Felix Eastcott and involved resecting the proximal internal and external carotid arteries. Mr. Eastcott then performed an internal carotid end to end anastomosis with the common carotid artery for reconstruction. The patient did well and was followed for 20 years. The operation was described in a famous paper by Eastcott, G. W. Pickering (who was the neurologist) and Rob in *The Lancet* in 1954. Three years later, Dr. Rob and H. B. Wheeler reported 27 more similar cases in the *British Medical Journal*. Subsequently, others have reported performing a carotid endarterectomy before 1954. In 1975 Michael DeBakey reported having performed a successful carotid endarterectomy in August, 1953. Dr. Rob estimates that he performed more than 5,000 carotid endarterectomy operations throughout his career.

Dr. Rob also pioneered the retro-peritoneal approach for abdominal aortic aneurysm repair. He presented a paper to the Society for Vascular Surgery that was subsequently published in the journal *Surgery* in 1963, outlining 500 patients treated in that way beginning with his first use of the approach in 1950.

After ten years leading at St. Mary's Hospital, Dr. Rob chose to move to the University of Rochester, in upstate New York, to become the chief of surgery there. Over the following 18 years, he built a prominent surgical department, including greatly advancing vascular surgery. Because of the University of Rochester's mandatory retirement age of 65, he accepted another job at East Carolina Medical School. Subsequently, at age 69, he was recruited by Norman Rich to Bethesda, Maryland to become a professor at the Uniformed Services University of Health Sciences.

Dr. Rob's unique career—coming at the very beginning of arterial surgery and spanning both sides of the Atlantic—gave him a truly worldwide perspective and personal acquaintance with nearly every pioneering vascular surgeon of the time. He was honored by being elected president of the International Cardiovascular Society in 1961. Ten years later, in 1971, he became president of the North American chapter of that group, which was called the International Society for Cardiovascular Surgery (NA-ISCVS). He was also honored to be a vice-president of the American Surgical Association in 1979. In 1975 the International Society of Surgery presented Dr. Rob with its René Leriche Prize.

Dr. Rob was also a prolific medical writer, and foremost of his accomplishments in that area is a set of eight volumes called *Operative Surgery* that he edited with Rodney Smith beginning in the mid-1950s. The set has since appeared in multiple editions.

As a young man, Charles Rob enjoyed skiing and mountaineering. He had four children and eight grandchildren. When he died at age 88, in Montpelier, Vermont, he was survived by his wife of 60 years, Mary Beasley Rob. They had been married during World War II, in 1941, when she was a nursing student at the Florence Nightingale Training School for Nurses at St. Thomas' Hospital, a few months before Dr. Rob headed to Tunisia with the paratroopers.

Scan the QR codes below or enter the YouTube links to watch both interviews with Dr. Charles Granville Rob conducted by Norman M. Rich on May 21, 1993 and June 18, 1993 in Bethesda, MD, as part of a historical video archive project, focusing particularly on military history, brought to you by the SVS History Project Work Group.p.

 Interview 1: https://tinyurl.com/RobXC8

 Interview 2: https://tinyurl.com/RobXC0

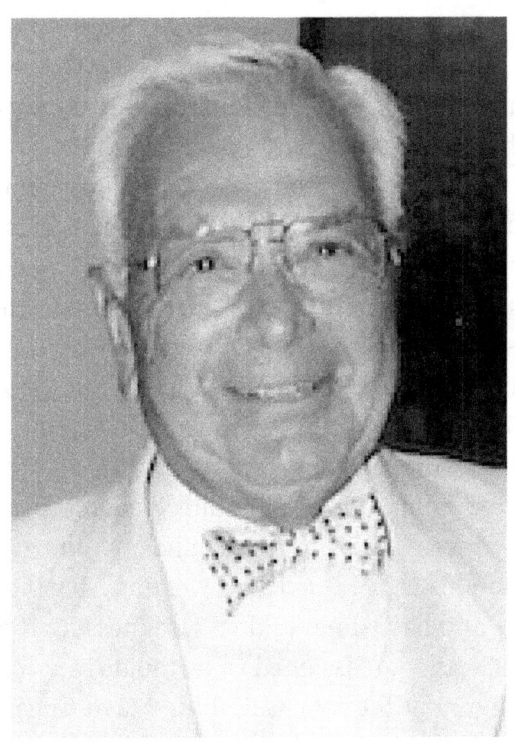

Harris B. Shumacker Jr., MD

Harris B. Shumacker was born on May 20, 1908 in Laurel, Mississippi and was raised and graduated from high school in Arkansas. He attended the University of Tennessee at Chattanooga for college where he took a very intense courseload and finished college after two years. Harris was accepted at Johns Hopkins for medical school, but decided to first spend a year at Vanderbilt University studying chemistry. He was awarded his MD degree at Johns Hopkins University in 1932 and was accepted to stay for his internship at Hopkins by Dean Dewitt Lewis, who was the surgical chairman at the time. Afterwards Shumacker worked in the surgical laboratory for two years at Johns Hopkins. His surgical training in general surgery was at Yale University.

After surgical training, Dr. Shumacker accepted a position as an instructor of surgery, first at Yale University from 1936 to 1938 and then back at Johns Hopkins. He had been at Hopkins for several years when Alfred Blalock was recruited from Vanderbilt University to be the new chief of surgery in 1941. In

1942 Dr. Shumacker joined the US Army and was assigned to the South Pacific theater of war, serving in Australia and then in New Guinea.

World War II had a pronounced effect on establishing vascular surgery as a separate entity. There were a large number of wounded soldiers with arterial-venous fistulas, traumatic false aneurysms, cold injury, and amputation from ligation of major blood vessels. To manage these individuals, the armed forces set up three vascular treatment centers in the United States, one of which was in Galesburg, Illinois, where a huge, 2,350-bed hospital complex was built in 1943. The unit was named the Mayo Army General Hospital after Charles and William Mayo, who had played a significant role with the Armed Forces during World War I. Just as this unit was being opened in the spring of 1944, Dr. Shumacker was being shipped back from the South Pacific where he had contracted a viral illness from which he had developed a perineal nerve injury and foot drop. There were no leg braces available in the war-zone, and he returned with a cast on his leg. He ended up wearing a leg brace on his right leg for about five years and had some residual weakness for the remainder of his life. Dr. Shumacker was soon assigned to be the director of the vascular center and chief of surgery at the new Galesburg Mayo General Army Hospital. He recalls having a single ward of 84 patients, all with arterial-venous fistulas and traumatic aneurysms requiring treatment. Injured patients were brought by railroad and delivered by a separate spurline built by the army directly to the hospital complex. Dr. Shumacker attributes his lifelong interest in vascular surgery to this experience.

When Dr. Shumacker was demobilized from the military in 1946, he returned to Yale as an associate professor of surgery. Soon afterwards, he was recruited to the Midwest and became the third chairman of the department of surgery at Indiana University Medical School in 1948. He served as chairman until 1968 establishing an outstanding surgical department, and becoming well known for his expertise and operative skill in the new fields of vascular and cardiovascular surgery. During his years as chairman, he continued to practice general surgery, all types of peripheral vascular, congenital heart, adult cardiac surgery, and surgery of the great vessels.

After he retired as chairman, Dr. Shumacker moved to a private practice setting at St. Vincent's Hospital in Indianapolis, establishing a cardiac surgery program there for nearly a decade. Later, Dr. Norman Rich recruited Dr. Shumacker to become a professor of surgery at the Uniformed Services University of Health Sciences in Bethesda, Maryland.

Dr. Shumacker's long distinguished career of surgical leadership and teaching includes membership and leadership of important surgical societies too numerous to detail. He produced over 600 articles and many chapters and several books including a very notable text, *The Evolution of Cardiac Surgery*, the first complete history of the development of heart surgery. It traces techniques from the ancient Greeks to the present day.

Dr. Shumacker's long affiliation with the Society for Vascular Surgery (SVS) began as one of the 31 founding members. At an organizational SVS meeting, held at the Fairmont Hotel in San Francisco on July 3, 1946, officers and chartered members were selected for the Society. He and Michael DeBakey, both 38 years old, were the youngest of the group. Dr. Shumacker served as treasurer of the SVS for the first six years beginning with the first official meeting on June 8, 1947, which was held at the Dennis Hotel in Atlantic City, New Jersey. He later served as the Society's 13th president from 1958 to 1959.

Likely, one of Dr. Shumacker's most important contributions to the SVS was writing an encyclopedic book entitled *The Society for Vascular Surgery: A History 1945 to 1983*. The excellence and importance of this highly readable 583-page book cannot be over emphasized. The 1984 copyright for the book is held by the Society for Vascular Surgery. It clearly outlines the dates and members present at the original organizational meetings, and then reviews the annual meetings themselves in detail with editorial comments on the most important papers. Dr. Shumacker prepared short biographies of all of the founding members, and also of all the Society presidents during the years up through 1983. He includes multiple appendices listing members, deceased members, officers, programs with the title of each paper and its authors from every annual program up through 1983, among many other references. One chapter, entitled "Antecedents" is a fascinating detailed history of advances in arterial and venous surgical technique from antiquity to the present.

Dr. Shumacker married Myrtle E. Landau in 1933. They were married for 58 years and had two sons and six grandchildren together. "Myrtie," as she was known, died in 1992 after which Dr. Shumacker married Grace. He died on November 14, 2009 at age 101 in Gladwyne, Pennsylvania.

Scan the QR code below or enter the YouTube link to watch the entire interview with Dr. Harris B. Shumacker conducted by Calvin B. Ernst, MD, brought to you by the SVS History Project Work Group.

 http://tinyurl.com/ShuXH

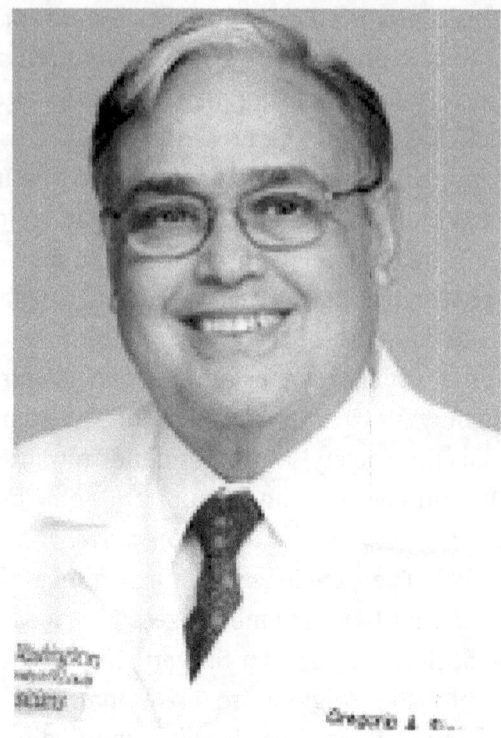

Gregorio A. Sicard, MD

Greg Sicard is well known for his national and international surgical leadership as well as for his role as chief of vascular surgery at the Washington University School of Medicine in St. Louis, Missouri. He was born on October 8, 1944 in Ponce, Puerto Rico but grew up in a smaller town 40 miles east called Guayama, a sugar processing area with four sugar mills. He is the son of a general surgeon father and a mother who was a nurse. Greg never had any doubt that surgery would be his medical specialty. He remembers his first visit to the operating room to watch his father operate when he was five years old, and there was never a time when he thought he would do anything else.

Greg's family arranged for him to complete his last year of high school in St. Louis, Missouri so that he could perfect his English. He ended up returning there for college at St. Louis University graduating in 1965. Greg went back to the University of Puerto Rico School of Medicine for his medical degree, graduating in 1972.

One of Greg's attendings in medical school was a close friend of Walter F. Ballinger II, who was the chief of surgery at Washington University in St. Louis. Therefore, Greg applied there and was accepted for his general surgery residency. An additional incentive for his return to the city was simple: St. Louis was the hometown of his college sweetheart and wife, with whom he now shares four children and numerous grandchildren.

After completing general surgery, Dr. Sicard stayed at Barnes Hospital, Washington University for a formal renal transplantation fellowship from 1977 to 1978. He then joined the surgical staff and practiced general, renal transplantation and vascular surgery. He soon established a tremendously busy clinical practice. His personal surgical volume reached 1,200 cases per year. He served as the section chief of vascular surgery from 1983 until 2012 and was also named the division chief of general surgery from 1998 to 2007.

Dr. Sicard developed an outstanding vascular fellowship, attracting talented applicants, some of whom he was able to hire to stay on his faculty. He also recruited vascular surgeons from outside, including Juan Parodi, who joined Dr. Sicard's group at Barnes Hospital for nearly three years. Dr. Parodi had been performing carotid artery stenting in Buenos Aires and was recruited, among other reasons, to teach the Washington University faculty that technique, which was completely new at the time.

Because of Dr. Sicard's great familiarity with retroperitoneal aortic area exposure from renal transplantation harvest procedures, he was a pioneer of this technique for aortic reconstruction. He routinely used the retroperitoneal exposure for both aortic occlusive and aortic aneurysm disease. In support of this approach he presented a very early paper comparing transabdominal and retroperitoneal aortic reconstruction to the Society for Vascular Surgery in 1986. Dr. Sicard was also an early adopter of aortic aneurysm endovascular technology. He initiated an innovative relationship with the private practice vascular surgeons in the St. Louis area, allowing them to have privileges at Barnes Hospital to be mentored on their own cases in order to develop aortic endovascular skills.

As a native Spanish speaker, Dr. Sicard frequently lectured on clinical and educational topics throughout Latin America and the Spanish-speaking world. Consequently, he became a prominent and respected leader not only in the United States but also abroad. Due to his organizational and leadership skills, Dr. Sicard was named president of many important surgical societies. He was the president of the American Association for Vascular Surgery in 2003–2004. Following this, he was president of the Society for Vascular Surgery from 2004 to 2005. Among his many honors and awards, Dr. Sicard received the René

Leriche Prize from the International Society of Surgery in 2017. For his many accomplishments and contributions to vascular surgery, the Society for Vascular Surgery awarded him its Lifetime Achievement Award in 2018.

Greg Sicard is a lifelong baseball fan and loves to golf. He is also an expert on fine cigars.

Scan the QR code below or enter the YouTube link to watch the entire interview with Dr. Gregorio A. Sicard conducted by Walter J. McCarthy, MD, brought to you by the SVS History Project Work Group.

 http://tinyurl.com/SicardXG

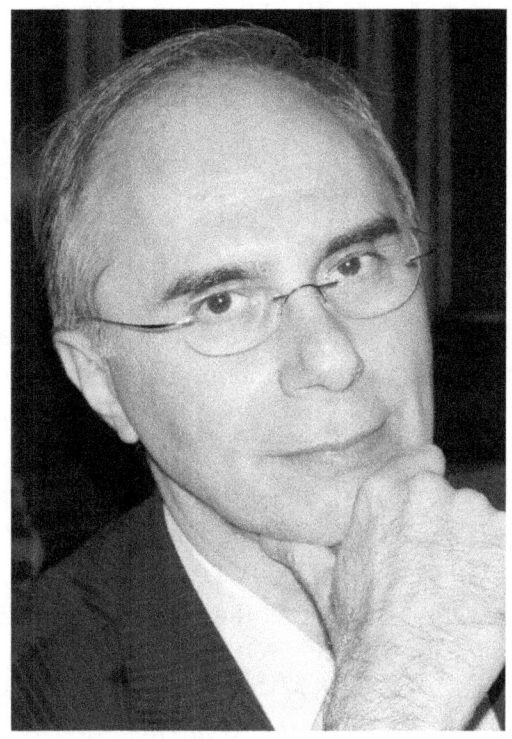

Anton N. Sidawy, MD

Anton Sidawy was born and raised in Damascus, Syria and attended medical school at Aleppo University School of Medicine in Aleppo, Syria. His parents had not had the opportunity to attend college and vigorously encouraged Tony, his two brothers and one sister toward higher education. His father taught the children French and English. Convinced that Tony should go into medicine, his father bought him medical books in English, including anatomy books and *Guyton's Physiology,* to read during high school. Being fluent in English and with many relatives living in Brooklyn, New York, Dr. Sidawy decided to come to the United States after he completed medical school. He completed general surgical training at Washington Hospital Center in Washington, DC. He and his wife had met earlier in medical school and were married during training. His wife eventually became the chief of surgical pathology at Georgetown University.

Years before, Dr. Sidawy had become interested in vascular surgery having read about it in *Time* magazine when Michael DeBakey was on the front cover. As a result, he sought vascular fellowships after general surgery training and was accepted at Boston University. He developed an understanding of what an academic vascular surgeon was during his fellowship at BU under the tutelage of important mentors, Frank LoGerfo and James Menzoian.

When Dr. Sidawy returned from Boston to Washington, DC, he became the chief of surgery at the Washington, DC, VA Medical Center, where he worked for 14 years. During that time he established a vascular fellowship and was the director for ten years. More recently, Dr. Sidawy has become Professor and the Lewis B. Saltz Chair of the Department of Surgery at George Washington University. Along the way he began taking courses in statistics, and eventually this evolved into a Master's Degree in Public Health with a concentration in medical administration from George Washington University.

Among his contributions to vascular surgery, Dr. Sidawy was the editor-in-chief of the *Journal of Vascular Surgery (JVS)* with his colleague Bruce Perler for more than seven years. During their time as editors, they established two sister journals for the *JVS*, one related to venous and lymphatic issues, and one for case reports. Dr. Sidawy has edited several surgical textbooks, including the ninth edition of *Rutherford's Vascular Surgery and Endovascular Surgery*, which was published in 2018. He has also published more than 180 papers and book chapters which reflect his early basic science experience and, more recently, his outcome and clinical research. Dr. Sidawy has been the president of several important vascular surgery societies including the Society for Vascular Surgery in 2010.

Dr. Sidawy has served on the Vascular Surgery Board of the American Board of Surgery and also as a Regent of the American College of Surgeons. In 2021, Dr. Sidawy was honored by being elected to the position of Chair of the American College of Surgeons Board of Regents.

Scan the QR code below or enter the YouTube link to watch the entire interview with Dr. Anton N. Sidawy conducted by William H. Baker, MD, and William H. Pearce, MD, brought to you by the SVS History Project Work Group.

 http://tinyurl.com/SidXA1

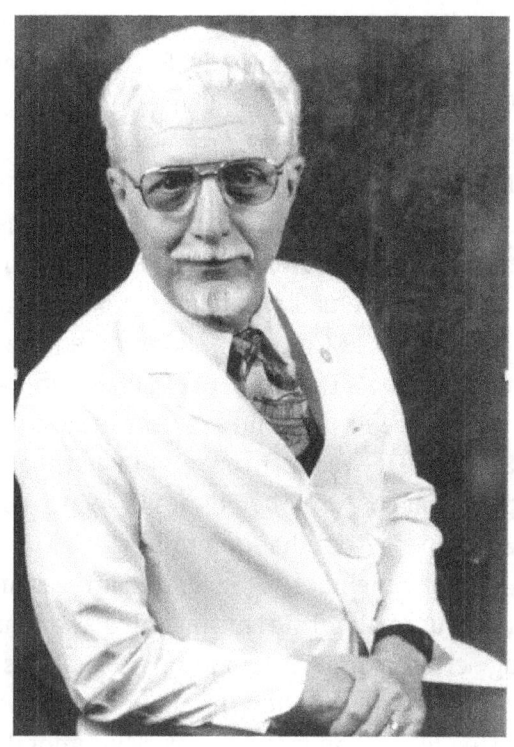

Robert B. Smith III, MD

Robert Smith was born on June 15, 1933. His parents had separated when he was an infant, and his mother remarried when he was seven years old. His mother, stepfather and the family lived with Bob's grandparents in a large house in Atlanta. Bob attended public school, was an Eagle Scout, and for college was admitted to Emory University on a scholarship. However, there were no scholarships offered for medical school at Emory. Fortunately, the pastor of the family's Methodist church arranged for an anonymous donor to pay Bob's tuition, and he was able to attend Emory University School of Medicine, where he graduated in 1957. He was honored with membership in the Phi Beta Kappa and AOA societies.

During his junior year in medical school Bob decided on surgery as a career path. After completing a surgical internship at Columbia Presbyterian Hospital in New York City, he served in the U.S. Army medical corps for two years, as was required for doctors at that time. He then completed his general surgery residency at Columbia Presbyterian during the time when Arthur Blakemore was chairman of the surgical department. Dr. Blakemore was a pioneer of the surgical treatment of portal hypertension using portocaval shunt surgery. At Columbia, Dr. Smith was also trained by Arthur Voorhees Jr., who became his lifelong mentor and friend. In 1953, Dr. Voorhees had fabricated and implanted the first prosthetic aortic bypass graft. He had done this using a Union Carbide synthetic cloth material called Vinyon-N. With this training background, a future in vascular surgery seemed preordained for Dr. Smith.

Dr. Smith finished training at Columbia, then joined the faculty of Emory University School of Medicine's Department of Surgery in 1966. He rose to the rank of Professor of Surgery in 1977 and served as the first John E. Skandalakis Professor of Surgery. He was instrumental in setting up one of the first vascular training programs in the United States in 1969, and he is very proud of the more than 60 trainees from that program.

Dr. Smith's bibliography includes 225 scientific articles and book chapters, and he has co-edited four textbooks. He is regarded as a master surgeon, and he estimates having performed more than 10,000 operations during his career. It is of interest that in 1977 he reported the first-ever axillary artery to popliteal artery bypass used to treat an infected aorto-bi-femoral graft. Besides his surgical and teaching responsibilities, over the years Dr. Smith held multiple administrative positions at Emory. These included being Chief of Surgical Services at the V.A. Medical Center, head of general vascular surgery, Associate Chairman of the Department of Surgery, Medical Director of Emory University Hospital, and Associate Dean for Clinical Services. His contributions and skills were also recognized by election to presidential leadership positions in multiple regional and national organizations, including the presidency of the North American Chapter of the International Society for Cardiovascular Surgery in 1996. For nearly a decade Dr. Smith served on the Board of Commissioners of the Joint Commission on Accreditation of Healthcare Organizations. For his many contributions to vascular surgery the Society for Vascular Surgery presented Dr. Smith with its Lifetime Achievement Award in 2020.

Dr. Smith retired in 2010 and lives in the Atlanta area with Flo, his wife of many years who he met in ninth grade.

Scan the QR code below or enter the YouTube link to watch the entire interview with Dr. Robert B. Smith III conducted by William H. Pearce, MD, and James S.T. Yao, MD, brought to you by the SVS History Project Work Group.

 http://tinyurl.com/SmithXR

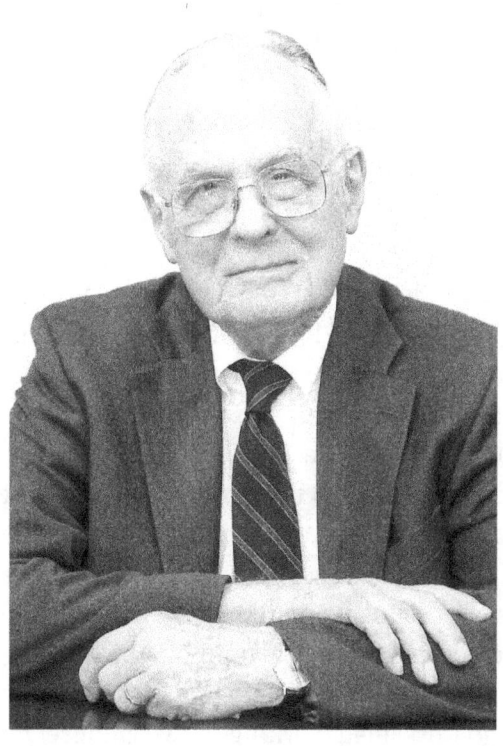

Frank C. Spencer, MD

Frank Cole Spencer was born in 1925 near the town of Haskell in north-central Texas. His grandfather had been a general practitioner, but his father did not attend college; instead, he had supported the family during the Great Depression as a farmer and rancher. Frank was homeschooled by his mother until third grade when he was able to attend a two-room school three miles from their farm. He rode his own pony to school and proved to be a very good student. For high school, Frank traveled by school bus seven miles each way and graduated at age 15 as the class valedictorian. He attended college at North Texas State University 150 miles east in Denton, Texas. Subsequently, both Texas medical schools rejected him because when he graduated from college he was only 17 years old. Fortunately, Vanderbilt University in Tennessee accepted his application, and he graduated in 1947 AOA.

Frank had his surgical training principally at Johns Hopkins Hospital in Baltimore, Maryland. This was interrupted by several years at UCLA, where he moved after his internship at Hopkins to train under William Longmire and then with service in the Korean War. Dr. Spencer had been deferred from the draft during World War II because he was in medical school, but he was called to pay this back and thus served in the Korean War from 1951 until 1953. He had committed himself to the U.S. Navy, which was assigning physicians to the Marine Corps during the Korean conflict. He served with the Marines in Easy Med Company near Panmunjom, Korea.

Although Dr. Spencer is remembered and eventually practiced as a cardiothoracic surgeon, likely his most important innovative contribution to surgery came from his combat experience repairing arteries in Korea. He later would say about this work, "arterial repair in Korea benefited more people than anything I've ever done." A unique aspect of the Korean War was that surgical treatment was occurring closer to the combat zone than it ever had before in history. Thanks to the proximity of the portable operating rooms to combat and the advent of helicopter transport, soldiers could be treated, sometimes within 30 minutes after being wounded.

Having had several years of surgical training, Dr. Spencer, who was 26 years old, was assigned to be the Chief of Surgery of a surgical unit staffed by eight other officers and 70 Corpsmen working in two Quonset huts. At the onset of the Korean conflict, related to vascular injury, orders were very clear that "all arterial injuries will be ligated." This was consistent with previous military surgical history. Not infrequently, this led to amputation, particularly of the lower extremity. Dr. Spencer was the only physician in the group trained to repair arteries having frequently been in the OR with Dr. Alfred Blalock during Blue Baby operations at Johns Hopkins during his internship. Blalock had first performed that operation, a left subclavian artery to left pulmonary artery anastomosis, in 1944 for tetralogy of Fallot. Dr. Spencer also had extensive animal laboratory experience and could confidently repair arteries. He made the decision to train all willing personnel to help with the surgery, realizing they risked court martial in doing so. All of the fellow surgeons joined in the effort. Equipment was sparse; initially there were only four bulldog serrafine vessel clamps. Rubber catheters were also used to occlude vessels. Eventually two Potts *ductus arteriosus* clamps arrived after six months, having been sent up to him by a colleague in southern Korea. Overall, the effort went very well, even by modern standards. Dr. Spencer's remarkable paper, *Ann Surg.* 1955 Mar; 141(3): 304–313, relates 89 arterial repairs with limb salvage of 95% for brachial, 79% for femoral and 62% for popliteal artery injuries. They used only local heparin irrigation, and 5–0 silk continuous suture, with a triangulation method based on Carrel's method. There were three vein grafts and 44 homografts which they obtained from autopsy material. At the conclusion of his service, Dr. Spencer received the Legion of Merit award and returned to Johns Hopkins to continue his residency. Years later, in 1978, he co-authored the classic book *Vascular Trauma* with Norman Rich, which included Dr. Rich's data from the Vietnam War.

Dr. Spencer's surgical career was always in universities: ten years at Johns Hopkins, four years in Kentucky and more than 40 years at NYU where he was Chairman of Surgery for 32 years. He has been honored as president of many major surgical organizations, among them the American Surgical Association (1997–1998), the American College of Surgeons (1990–1991), the American Association of Thoracic Surgery (1982–1983)—which presented him a Lifetime Achievement Award in 2010, and the International Society for Cardiovascular Surgery. He is remembered for his great enthusiasm for surgery, his talent for leadership, his love and dedication to teaching and his tremendous work ethic.

Dr. Spencer died on July 23, 2018 at the age of 92.

Scan the QR code below or enter the YouTube link to watch the entire interview with Dr. Frank C. Spencer conducted by Roger T. Gregory, MD, brought to you by the SVS History Project Work Group.

 http://tinyurl.com/SpencerXF

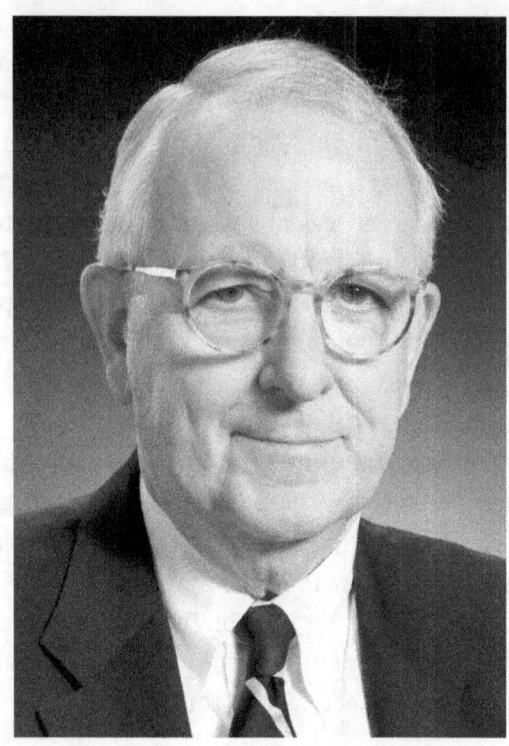

James C. Stanley, MD

James C. Stanley is Professor Emeritus of Surgery at the University of Michigan, the institution from which he received his medical degree in 1964. Jim had grown up in East Lansing, Michigan and originally intended to become an automotive engineer. He had restored a 1932 Plymouth car while in high school, and his career plan was engineering school followed by a degree in metallurgy at MIT! But during engineering school at Michigan, Jim read several books by the physician and humanitarian author Tom Dooley, about work in southeast Asia. As a result, he was inspired to change course to medicine as a career. Michigan was the obvious choice. After that, following his internship at Philadelphia General Hospital, he served as a medical officer at the Brooke Army Center before completing his surgical residency at the University of Michigan.

It is not surprising that Dr. Stanley chose vascular surgery for his career. He remembers that during his surgical residency he spent eleven months of training on the service of C. Gardner Child, who was the surgical chairman and is remembered as a pioneer portocaval shunt surgeon. At Michigan, he was also taught and mentored by Bill DeWeese, who had performed the world's first aortorenal bypass, and Bill Fry, a vascular surgery pioneer.

Dr. Stanley joined the faculty of his *alma mater* where he eventually served as the head of the Vascular Surgery Section from 1976–2004. During that tenure, one of eight of the nation's program directors in vascular surgery was trained at the University of Michigan. He was the Director of the Jobst Vascular Research Laboratories from 1989–2004 and was a Director of the University's Cardiovascular Center from 2003–2014. Specializing in all areas of vascular surgery, Dr. Stanley's clinical practice has specifically focused on renovascular hypertension, splanchnic aneurysms and pediatric arterial diseases. He is a world authority related to pediatric renovascular hypertension and renal artery bypass in children. He has always maintained an ongoing interest in biomedical research and received an NIH Vascular Disease Academic Award in 1993. Dr. Stanley was the recipient of the Michigan Medical Center Alumni Distinguished Achievement Award in 2000, and the medical school's Lifetime Achievement Award in Clinical Care in 2014.

Dr. Stanley has given more than 700 presentations in the United States and abroad. He is an honorary fellow of the Royal College of Surgeons, Edinburgh, an honorary member of the Academy of Medicine of Columbia and the Royal Australasian College of Surgeons, Section of Vascular. In addition, Dr. Stanley has served as president of numerous learned societies including the Society for Vascular Surgery, 1996–1997, an organization that granted him its Lifetime Achievement Award in 2012. He has authored more than 550 scientific articles and textbook chapters, and he served as the editor of *The Journal of Vascular Surgery* from 1991 until 1996. Dr. Stanley has edited 15 books, including two on renovascular hypertension, one on biologic and synthetic vascular prostheses, and five editions of *Current Therapy in Vascular Surgery*.

Dr. Stanley has been married for more than 50 years, and he and his wife raised three children. He is an avid lepidopterist, a novice marathon runner and a devotee of classical and improvisational jazz music. He has recently written three memoirs.

Scan the QR code below or enter the YouTube link to watch the entire interview with Dr. James C. Stanley conducted by Walter J. McCarthy, MD, and James S.T. Yao, MD, brought to you by the SVS History Project Work Group.

 http://tinyurl.com/StanleyXJ

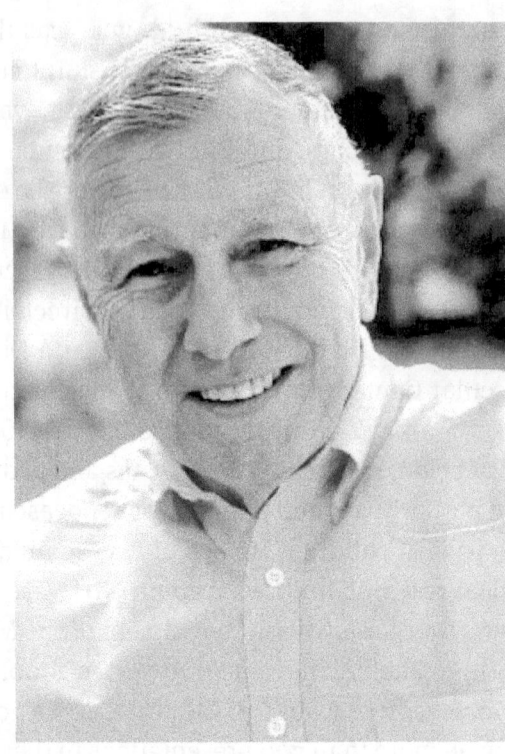

Ronald J. Stoney, MD

Ronald Stoney was born and grew up in Carmel, California. His father worked as a carpenter and building contractor and his mother as a seamstress. Carmel was very rural when Ron was born on March 4, 1934, and he remembers a boyhood of outdoor activities, hunting, ranching and farming. Ron was inspired toward biology by a high school teacher, and later biology was his major when he graduated from nearby Santa Clara University in 1955.

The University of California San Francisco (UCSF) was an obvious choice for medical school. After graduating in 1959, Dr. Stoney completed a rotating internship at the San Francisco General Hospital followed by a general surgery residency at UCSF (1960–1965). At UCSF Dr. Stoney was taught and mentored by the pioneer vascular surgeon, Edwin "Jack" Wylie, with whom he would eventually practice. Dr. Wylie is credited with establishing the very first vascular surgery fellowship in the United States at UCSF in 1962. It is of interest that when the American Board of Surgery began issuing certificates of "Special

Competency in General Vascular Surgery" in 1982, Dr. Wylie was issued certificate number one.

In 1962, with Malcolm Perry as Dr. Wylie's first fellow, Dr. Stoney was the second-year general surgery resident on their service. Several years later, Dr. Stoney also completed his vascular surgery fellowship at UCSF and then was asked by Dr. Wylie and the Chief of Surgery, Dr. J. Engelbert Dunphy, to join the faculty. The very next year, after graduating from the fellowship, William Ehrenfeld also joined the vascular practice. Their surgical group, referred to as Wylie, Stoney and Ehrenfeld, established an iconic vascular surgery practice that was known worldwide and set new standards of excellence in surgical care and training.

Dr. Stoney became recognized for developing innovative solutions to difficult surgical problems, including re-operations and particularly very complex aortic occlusive and aneurysmal disease involving the viscera. Related to these interests, during a four-month sabbatical in Australia in 1980, Dr. Stoney observed a rudimentary self-retaining retractor. He borrowed the instrument to help during the repair of a renal artery aneurysm he performed while in Australia. He was impressed by the more stable surgical exposure provided compared with hand-held retractors. After returning to the United States, he worked with an engineer colleague to develop a practical self-retaining retractor system. They literally began work in a two-car garage on their project. This eventually resulted in a side-rail, operating-table-mounted device. First called a Stoney Retractor, it is now known as the Omni-Tract retractor. This device is used throughout the world, not only by vascular surgeons but also by surgeons of many other specialties.

Known as a gifted technical surgeon, Dr. Stoney always remained dedicated to teaching and research. He was involved in training hundreds of students, residents and more than 70 vascular fellows, including many who have become leaders at centers around the world. He has contributed several hundred publications and co-authored nine books, emphasizing the operative approach, the disease itself and the technical maneuvers required to achieve safe, effective and durable outcomes for patients. The best-known of these textbooks is the two-volume *Manual of Vascular Surgery*. These two large-format books, with beautiful color illustrations, make available to other surgeons much of the vast vascular surgical experience developed at the UCSF.

In 1982, Dr. Stoney co-founded the Pacific Vascular Research Foundation, now called Vascular Cures, which supports the career development of promising young vascular surgeons and invests in basic technology aimed at improving treatments that enhance human health.

Among his many honors, Dr. Stoney was named the fourth president of the Western Vascular Society in 1990 and also president of the North American Chapter of the International Society for Cardiovascular Surgery. For his many contributions, the Society for Vascular Society granted Dr. Stoney its second Lifetime Achievement Award in 2006. Having retired from clinical practice in 2000, currently Dr. Stoney is Emeritus Professor of Surgery at UCSF, where he continues to teach surgery residents and perform clinical research.

Scan the QR code below or enter the YouTube link to watch the entire interview with Dr. Ronald J. Stoney conducted by Norman M. Rich, MD, brought to you by the SVS History Project Work Group.

 http://tinyurl.com/StoneyXR

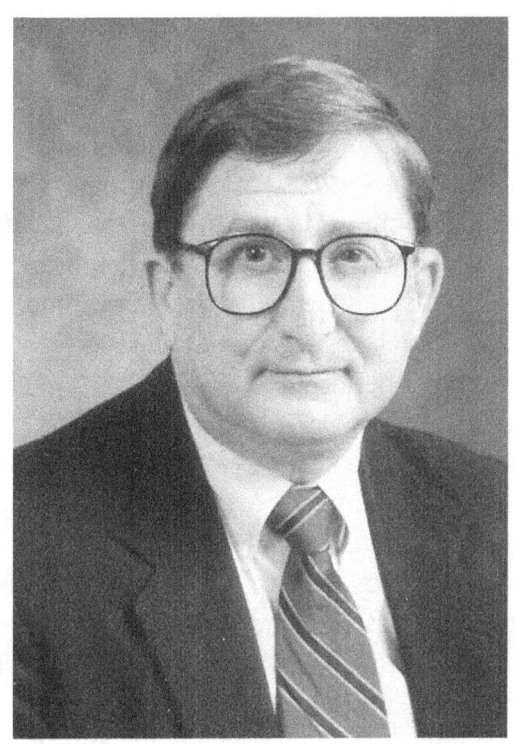

Jonathan B. Towne, MD

Jonathan Towne was born and raised in Youngstown, Ohio. After high school, he attended the University of Pittsburgh, graduating in 1963. Jon was hospitalized briefly while in college during which time he followed the course of a nearby patient who had had a femoral-popliteal bypass for gangrene. Jon also met the patient's vascular surgeon. He was fascinated by what he had seen and decided what he hoped his career would be. After college, Jon attended the University of Rochester School of Medicine and Dentistry, graduating in 1967. Having selected surgery, his PGY I and PGY II years were at the University of Michigan, where he met and operated with the pioneer vascular surgeon, William Fry. Jon finished general surgery at the University of Nebraska. He had elected to defer his mandatory military service through the Berry Plan until after completing his surgical training. Consequently, in 1972–1974 he served as the Chief of General Surgery at Vanderberg Air Force Base near Santa Maria, California. During the Vietnam War, normally the second half of these two years would have been spent operating somewhere in Vietnam, but by 1974 any young surgeons who were fathers were not being sent to the war zone.

Following his military service, Dr. Towne completed a one-year vascular surgery fellowship at Baylor University Hospital in Dallas, Texas. The fellowship was under the direction of Dr. Jesse Thompson, who had established one of the first vascular training programs in the United States in 1964. One of the earliest practitioners of carotid surgery, Dr. Thompson was truly a master carotid artery surgeon. He had performed the first carotid endarterectomy in Dallas in 1957. With this tutelage, Dr. Towne still rates carotid endarterectomy as his favorite operation to perform.

After his vascular fellowship, Dr. Towne was recruited to Milwaukee in 1975 by Victor Bernhard and for the next 33 years was on the faculty of the Medical College of Wisconsin in Milwaukee. Dr. Towne co-authored a superb, definitive textbook with Dr. Bernhard called *Complications in Vascular Surgery*, which they published in 1980. The text has since been re-issued in multiple editions. Dr. Towne served as the Chief of Vascular Surgery and also taught young surgeons, including 29 fellows, and directed the vascular fellowship at the Medical College of Wisconsin for many years. Some of his most important published research has involved hypercoagulation and also prosthetic bypass graft infection, particularly related to *Staphylococcus aureus*.

Dr. Towne has been honored with multiple important national leadership roles. These include being a director of the American Board of Surgery, president of the Central Surgical Association (2002–2003) and president of the Society for Vascular Surgery (1999–2000), which in 2022 granted Dr. Towne its Lifetime Achievement Award in Boston. Dr. Towne retired on July 27, 2012 as Emeritus Professor of Surgery. In 2007 Dr. Towne was honored by his department with an annual visiting professorship in his name.

Dr. Towne married Sandra Jean Green on August 24, 1963. They have three children, Tim, Heidi and Crista, and multiple grandchildren. He now lives in Carbondale, Colorado.

Scan the QR code below or enter the YouTube link to watch the entire interview with Dr. Jonathan B. Towne conducted by Walter J. McCarthy, MD, brought to you by the SVS History Project Work Group.

 https://tinyurl.com/TowneXJ2

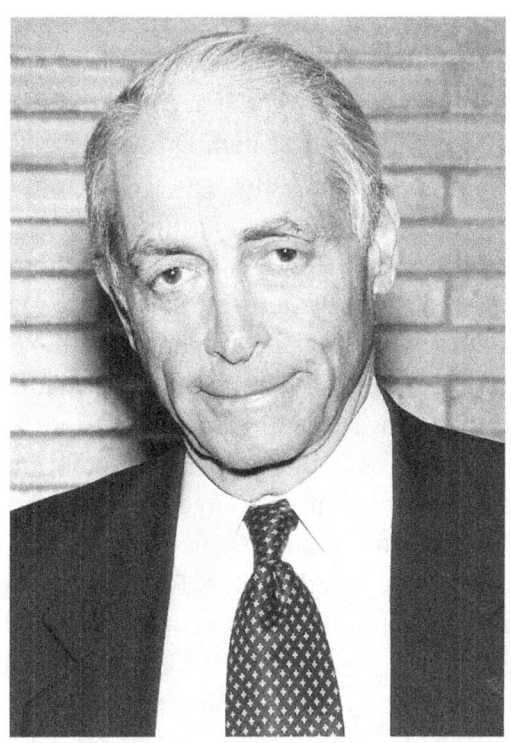

Frank J. Veith, MD

Frank J. Veith is a New York City vascular surgeon, leader of vascular surgeons and surgical innovator. He is recognized worldwide by vascular surgeons for his outstanding annual teaching conference in New York City, often accompanied by a bound or virtual textbook. This conference, termed the VEITH Symposium, is in its 48th year as of 2021. At its peak, as many as 5000 attendees visited this meeting each year

Dr. Veith has been the president of many important vascular surgery societies, including the Society for Vascular Surgery from 1995 to 1996. His national leadership included an ardent, hard-fought campaign to establish a separate board for vascular surgery in the United States distinct from the American Board of Surgery. The concept of a separate vascular board was supported by the majority of practicing vascular surgeons at that time. Dr. Veith helped establish and was the Chairman of the American Board of Vascular Surgery. This new board however, was ultimately denied by the American Board of Medical Specialties.

Frank Veith was born in New York City, August 29, 1931. His mother was a registered nurse of Irish descent, and his father was an attorney of German descent. Frank's great-grandfather Veith had come to the United States at age 14 and became a successful businessman. Dr. Veith was an only child who attended a private high school and then graduated from Cornell University, Phi Beta Kappa, in 1952.

He attended Cornell University for medical school where he graduated first in his class in 1955. After a surgical internship at Columbia-Presbyterian in New York City, the remainder of his surgical training was at the Peter Bent Brigham Hospital in the Harvard system in Boston. At the Brigham, Dr. Veith served under Francis Moore, who was the Chief of Surgery. He was also trained by Dwight Harken and considers both surgeons important mentors. During residency, he conducted transplantation-related surgical research under Joseph Murray, who had performed a kidney transplant between identical twins in 1954. Murray eventually received the Nobel Prize for that work in 1990.

During Dr. Veith's surgical training, after the fourth year, he entered the military through the Berry Plan. He served in the U.S. Army as a captain and chief of the surgical service at Fort Carson in Colorado Springs, Colorado (1960–62) after which he returned to Boston to complete his residency.

Returning home to New York City as a young attending, Dr. Veith worked for a short time at Cornell and Bellevue Hospitals. Soon afterwards, he moved to Albert Einstein Medical College and Montefiore Medical Center in the Bronx, where he remained for his entire clinical career. There he was initially named the Chief of Transplant Surgery, performing kidney transplants and also beginning pioneering work in lung transplantation. He also performed a considerable amount of vascular surgery and was named Chief of Vascular Surgery in 1972. Later, Dr. Veith became the Chairman of Surgery at Montefiore and Albert Einstein College of Medicine.

Dr. Veith's career encompassed all types of vascular surgery. Faced with large numbers of patients with lower extremity limb-threatening arterial disease in his early career, many of his publications centered on lower extremity bypass. In the 1970s, Dr. Veith was among the very first to advocate for an aggressive approach to limb salvage with arterial bypass, including using prosthetic grafts to reach tibial arteries.

Dr. Veith later performed and reported the first repair of an abdominal aortic aneurysm using endovascular techniques in North America. This important accomplishment was performed together with Juan Parodi and Claudio Schonholz from Argentina and the New York City vascular surgeon, Michael Marin, at Montefiore Hospital in November, 1992. After this Dr. Veith became a leading proponent of the endovascular stent graft technique for both elective and particularly also for ruptured aortic aneurysms.

Besides his distinguished leadership, clinical surgery and symposium-directing activities, Dr. Veith has also published more than 1000 peer-reviewed vascular surgery-related articles and ten textbooks. For these many important accomplishments guiding vascular surgery, he has been recognized with career achievement awards by many national and international societies including the Society for Vascular Surgery's Lifetime Achievement Award in 2010.

Scan the QR code below or enter the YouTube link to watch the entire interview with Dr. Frank J. Veith conducted by Roger T. Gregory, MD, brought to you by the SVS History Project Work Group.

 Interview 1: http://tinyurl.com/VeithXF1

 Interview 2: http://tinyurl.com/VeithXF2

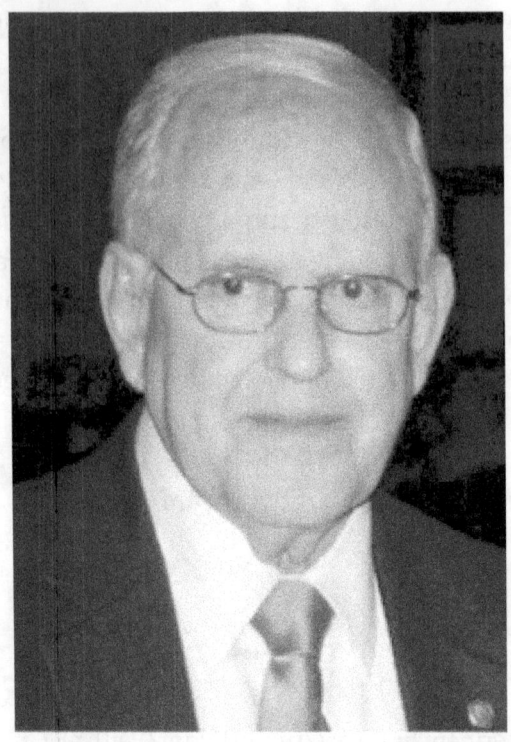

J. Leonel Villavicencio, MD

Leonel Villavicencio was born in Mexico City, Mexico on August 8, 1926, the oldest of six children. He grew up in Sonora, a region in northern Mexico. His father was a colonel in the Mexican army and taught him to shoot and took him hunting. Leonel's father, a heavy smoker, developed a "pulmonary condition" and died in 1941. This left the family very financially stressed with his mother working at the post office to support the children.

Leonel's college education was at the National University of Mexico. During college Leonel did very well on the medical school entry exams and was able to be admitted to the military medical school where the education was tuition-free. He thus became a military doctor. Leonel attended the Hospital Central Militar for surgical training in general surgery. Afterwards he was able to obtain a scholarship for further training outside of Mexico. He came to Chicago in 1956, to the University of Illinois, for a year of vascular fellowship under Professor Geza de Takats. In Chicago, he was also taught and mentored by the pioneer arterial surgeons Ormand Julian, William Sam Dye and Hushang Javid. Dr. de Takats helped him arrange an interview in Boston, and subsequently he spent several training years in Boston devoted to vascular surgery with Richard Warren and Robert Linton. This was followed by two years of cardiac surgery under Dwight Harkin at the Brigham Hospital and Dr. Robert Gross at Children's in Boston. There he met his wife, who was a nurse in the ICU at Children's Hospital.

The newly married couple returned to Mexico City in 1962 where Dr. Villavicencio became the only cardiovascular surgeon in a 1000-bed hospital. He performed open heart surgery, venous surgery, arterial bypasses and amputations. He recalls performing the then-innovative technique of in-situ saphenous vein bypass starting in 1966.

Dr. Villavicencio was named Chief of Surgery at the Army Hospital in Mexico City and Vice-Chairman at the Children's Hospital, performing open heart surgery for children. He later became president of the Mexican Society of Vascular Surgery and also president of the Mexican chapter of the American College of Surgeons.

As department chairman, Dr. Villavicencio invited Dr. Norman Rich from Walter Reed Hospital to Mexico to be a visiting professor, and they subsequently became friends. Through this friendship, an opportunity eventually came for Dr. Villavicencio and his wife to move to the United States, when he accepted a position at the Uniformed Services School of Medicine, Walter Reed Army Medical Center in July, 1983. At Walter Reed he established the very first teaching clinic in the military for venous and lymphatic diseases in 1984. He directed the clinic for 20 years. After moving to Washington, Dr. Villavicencio stopped performing cardiac surgery and concentrated entirely on vascular surgery. Always interested in venous problems, he focused in that area. It is noteworthy that he was one of the original founders of the American Venous Forum in 1989.

Dr. Villavicencio passed away on January 14, 2019.

Scan the QR code below or enter the YouTube link to watch the entire interview with Dr. J. Leonel Villavicencio conducted by Roger T. Gregory, MD, brought to you by the SVS History Project Work Group.

 http://tinyurl.com/VillaXL

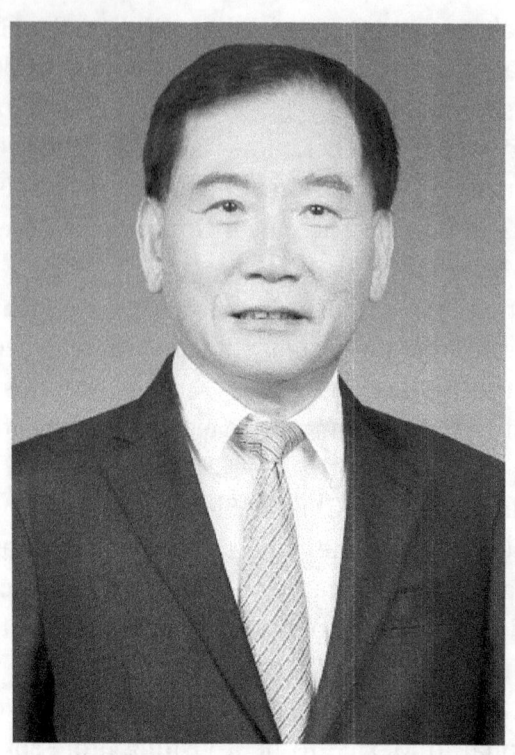

Shenming Wang, MD, PhD

Shenming Wang, MD, PhD, FACS, is an academic leader and Chief of Vascular Surgery at the First Affiliated Hospital of Sun Yat-sen University in southern China. He is also the Honorary Leader of the Vascular Surgery Group of the Chinese Medical Association. In 2013, Professor Wang served as the president of the Chinese Society for Vascular Surgery, which has a restricted membership of only 40 national vascular surgery leaders. Professor Wang has also been president of the Chinese Association for Phlebology of the International Union of Phlebology, president of the Asian Venous Forum and is an honorary member of the Society for Vascular Surgery. He is Director of the Engineering Research Center for the Diagnosis and Treatment of Vascular Diseases in Guangdong and Director of the National Local Joint Engineering Laboratory of the Diagnosis and Treatment of Vascular Diseases in Guangdong.

Professor Wang has served as the Chief Editor of the *Chinese Journal of Vascular Surgery,* the *Chinese Journal of Vascular Surgery* (Electronic Edition) and of the *Chinese Archives of General Surgery* (Electronic Edition). He is the Deputy Editor of the *Chinese Medical Journal* and many other core journals.

Dr. Wang and his wife—who works in the import/export business—have a single child as stipulated by the "one-child policy" of the People's Republic of China at the time. Dr. Wang is from a medical family that includes at least four generations: His grandfather was a practitioner of traditional Chinese medicine, his mother a pediatrician, his father a surgeon, and his son a urologist who received training at Yale in New Haven, Connecticut.

Dr. Wang began his medical education in 1977, just at the end of the "cultural revolution," which had come to a close with Chairman Mao's death the year before. He graduated in medicine in 1982, had completed his Masters and PhD by 1989, and by 1997 was a full professor of surgery. An important part of Dr. Wang's training occurred at the University of Pittsburgh during 1996 and 1997. He had been invited there by the master liver transplant surgeon, Professor Thomas Starzl, and began studying liver anatomy and vascular anastomotic technique with him. Dr. Wang was drawn to vascular surgery by the "skill, technique and challenge" of the specialty. Therefore, he also spent eight months in Pittsburgh under the tutelage of Marshall Webster, who was chief of vascular surgery. Dr. Wang was exposed to the traditional open methods of carotid endarterectomy, aortic aneurysm repair and lower extremity prosthetic and vein bypass during those months.

Eventually Dr. Wang became the director of vascular surgery of a 4000-bed hospital in the city of Guangzhou, China, which is located 75 miles northwest of Hong Kong. Previously called Canton, Guangzhou is a city of 19 million. Dr. Wang's unit includes 20 vascular surgeons, and he recalls that endovascular treatment of the aorta began in 2000. Interestingly, his unit published a series of 215 cases of thoracic aorta endovascular repair in the *Journal of Vascular Surgery* in 2008. All of the cases were done with Gore-Tex devices and, most notably, some had the proximal landing zone in the ascending aorta, if there was room above the aortic valve and the coronary artery orifices. At the time of his interview, on June 1, 2017, Dr. Wang estimated that his unit had performed about 500 "endo" repairs for type-B dissections and that they generally treated even uncomplicated type-B cases with stent-grafts.

Scan the QR code below or enter the YouTube link to watch the entire interview with Dr. Shenming Wang conducted by Walter J. McCarthy, MD, and Jinsong Wang, MD, brought to you by the SVS History Project Work Group.

 http://tinyurl.com/WangXS

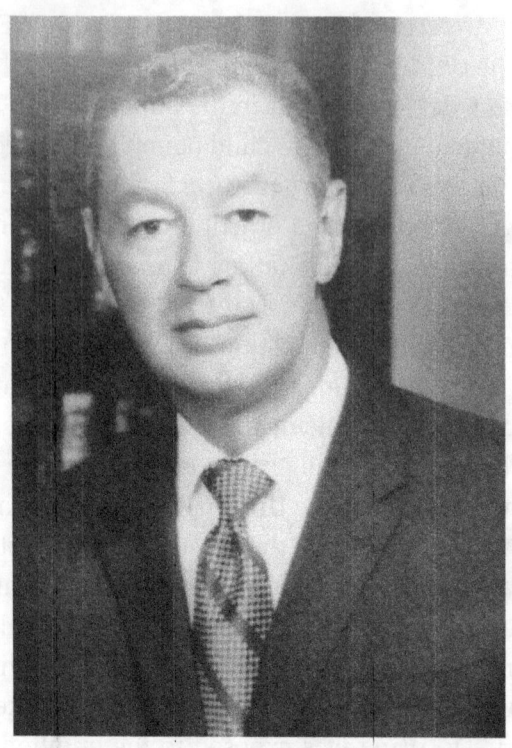

Milton Weinberg, MD

Milton Weinberg was born in the small farming community of Sumter, South Carolina in August, 1924. His father was a urologist who had graduated from Johns Hopkins Medical School in 1914. After Milton finished high school in 1941, he attended college at Duke University. Milton also went to medical school at Duke, graduating in 1946. He considered going into pediatrics, but after studying surgery during his final rotation, his mind was set on becoming a surgeon.

Before beginning his surgical internship at Duke, he did a six-month interim surgical internship at the Church Home and Infirmary in Baltimore. After his time at Duke, Dr. Weinberg then went to Charleston, South Carolina for another year of internship and eventually finished his general surgery residency there. However, the Korean War, which started in June 1950, interrupted his residency.

He was inducted into the Army on January 1, 1951 at Fort Sam Houston,

Texas and was in Korea nine days later. Dr. Weinberg served initially in a clearing company, just behind the combat troops, evaluating and prepping the wounded before moving them back by ambulance for more advanced care. In June of 1951, he was transferred to the 8055 MASH unit. The Mobile Army Surgical Hospital was a concept invented during World War II by Dr. DeBakey and the Surgical Consultants to bring surgical care closer to the front-line. In Korea, MASH units were comprised of three tents with wooden flooring for housing, storage and surgery. The unit could move forward or backward to stay within 7–15 miles of the fighting. Dr. Weinberg's outfit received as many as 1,000 casualties a day. The wounded were typically transported by ambulances, but their unit also had three helicopters. Dr. Weinberg said the vast majority of injuries he treated were from shell fragments which tore tissue. Thus, many of the operations were debridements. The surgeons put in chest tubes but rarely opened the chest as most such injuries would have been fatal at the scene. They had all of the equipment and fresh blood that they needed. There were many abdominal injuries requiring bowel and renal surgery, however, Dr. Weinberg remembers only a few extremity amputations and no vessel repairs. While Dr. Weinberg later enjoyed the film version of the *M*A*S*H* franchise, he disliked the television show because he felt it belittled the regular army personnel—whom he came away greatly respecting. He left Korea at age 28 and said he was "little bit more serious and a little bit older" as a surgeon.

After being discharged in 1952, Dr. Weinberg returned to Charleston and finished there as chief surgical resident. Under his mentors, Drs. Fred Cradle and Edward Parker, he learned a great deal about thoracic and cardiac procedures. He worked on lung resections and assisted in Hufnagle valve procedures. The remarkable Hufnagle operation involved placing a ball-valve device quickly within the cross-clamped and opened descending aorta as a treatment for severe aortic valve insufficiency. These procedures were the very first prosthetic heart valve operations and did not require cardiopulmonary bypass.

Dr. Weinberg came to Chicago in July of 1955 and worked informally with Dr. Egbert Fell who practiced at both Presbyterian Hospital and Cook County Hospital. This was the era of the very beginning of the heart-lung machine and the bubble oxygenator. One of Dr. Weinberg's assignments was to be the assistant director of the Chicago Artery Bank, which had been established by Dr. Fell in 1955. The Bank, initially housed at the Hektoen Institute adjacent to Cook County Hospital, freeze-dried aortic homografts obtained from autopsy rooms across the city. The aortic grafts were stored in sterile glass tubes and re-hydrated with saline in the OR for use as arterial bypasses and for other repairs. Dr. Weinberg's paper summing up this experience describes more than 300 cases performed by surgeons in Chicago over a three year period. The advent of fabric grafts in the mid-to-late 1950s replaced the need for these homografts.

Presbyterian and St. Luke's Hospitals merged in 1958. During this time, Dr. Weinberg worked with Dr. Fell and side-by-side with the pioneer vascular and cardiac surgeons Ormand Julian, Husang Javid and Sam Dye. In 1964 he was invited by Drs. Robert Freeark and Robert Baker to develop the first thoracic residency program at Cook County Hospital, and he remembers Dr. Thomas Murphy as his first trainee. Dr. Weinberg was Chairman of the Department of Cardio-Thoracic Surgery at Cook County Hospital between 1964 and 1968.

Dr. Weinberg retired as a surgeon after 31 years at Rush, where he had also served as President of the Medical Staff and a member of the Board of Trustees (1977–1979) when he was 65 years old. He then accepted another Chicago position and became the Chair of Surgery at Lutheran General Hospital in 1987.

In retirement Dr. Weinberg lives with Joan, his wife of many years, and enjoys photography. He said he considers himself to know something about nursing, since first his mother, then his wife and two of their three daughters are nurses.

Scan the QR code below or enter the YouTube link to watch the entire interview with Dr. Milton Weinberg conducted by Walter J. McCarthy, MD, John V. White, MD, and James S.T. Yao, MD, brought to you by the SVS History Project Work Group.

 http://tinyurl.com/WeinbergXM

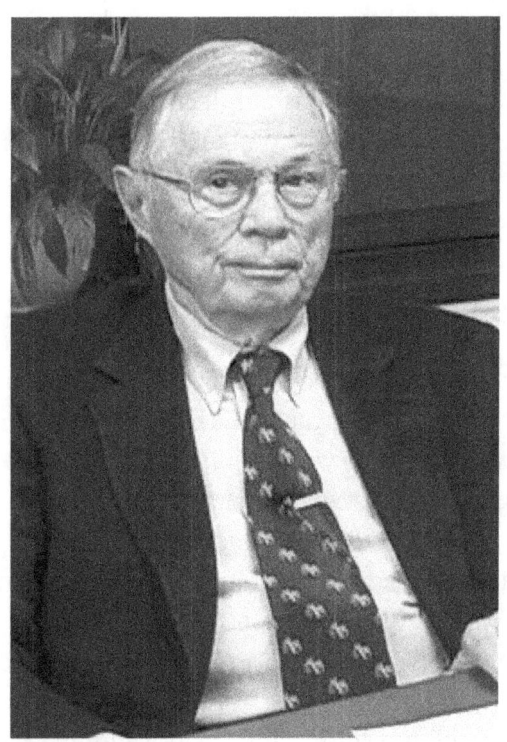

Jock R. Wheeler, MD

Jock R. Wheeler was born in September 1932 and was raised in Hampton, Virginia. He graduated from Hampton High School in 1950 and matriculated to Virginia Military Institute, graduating in 1954 wearing academic stars. Dr. Wheeler attended the Medical College of Virginia (now Virginia Commonwealth University) and stayed to complete his surgical training under Dr. David Hume, who had recently arrived from Boston to be the chief of surgery. Dr. Hume was a pioneer renal transplant surgeon who had been with Dr. Joseph Murray in 1954 when their team performed the world's first successful human kidney transplant. Dr. Hume was also very interested in vascular surgery, and Jock remembers many aortic aneurysm repairs with Dacron grafts and also some aorto-bi-femoral and femoral-popliteal bypasses during his general surgical training.

Following completion of his internship, Dr. Wheeler was commissioned in the U.S. Navy as a Lieutenant. He served for three years as a flight surgeon, traveling with a Marine fighter squadron to a number of locations, including Guantanamo Bay during the Bay of Pigs invasion in 1961.

After Dr. Wheeler returned to finish his residency following military service, Dr. Hume arranged an NIH postdoctoral fellowship for him to study with Sir Roy Calne at Westminster Hospital in London in the field of Transplant & Immunology. Professor Calne was also a pioneer transplant surgeon and had been a fellow with Dr. Murray in Boston. Sir Peter Medawar, who had received the Nobel Prize in Medicine in 1958, was also part of his educational experience in England. Five publications in the *British Journal of Medicine* came from this work: two first-authored by Dr. Wheeler, the other three authored by Calne, Medawar, Wheeler *et al.* Dr. Wheeler greatly enjoyed the year in London with his wife and three young children. He remembers not only transplant surgery, large animal transplant surgery involving baboons, and also a considerable amount of vascular surgery. On one interesting occasion he had the privilege of staffing the first-aid station for the lying in state of Sir Winston Churchill at Westminster Hall in 1965.

After finishing his surgical residency in 1966, Dr. Wheeler chose Norfolk, Virginia to start his surgical practice. The need for a medical school in this region had been identified and the start of the Eastern Virginia Medical School was underway. Soon afterward, in 1970, the Kidney Transplant Program at Norfolk General Hospital was established, with Dr. Wheeler performing the first kidney transplant there in 1972. Three years later the vascular surgery fellowship was established by Dr. Wheeler and Dr. Roger Gregory. It was one of twenty vascular fellowship programs in the country at that time, and Dr. Wheeler was the program director from 1975 until 1994. Today, this fellowship is in its forty-fourth year of training vascular surgeons.

In 1975, Dr. Wheeler was involved with the first successful human Gore-Tex polytetraflouroethylene (PTFE) femoral-popliteal bypass. He assisted his junior partner, Roger Gregory, with the operation on August 25, 1975 for a semi-emergent femoral to below popliteal reconstruction for limb salvage to help a woman who had had both saphenous veins previously removed. Dr. Gregory had heard about the product and had called Gore-Tex the day before. The phone had been answered by Jack Hoover. Mr. Hoover, who became the company's legendary sales representative, flew all night to get the 6 mm graft from Flagstaff, Arizona to Norfolk. The operation went well and utilized 5-0 prolene suture. The needle holes bled "like a watering pot" but came under control after reversing the heparin. Sometime later the two surgeons learned that they had been the first to ever use the Gore-Tex graft!

Besides his busy clinical practice and surgical teaching, Dr. Wheeler held a number of major administrative and leadership positions. He served as president of the Southern Association for Vascular Surgery in 1999. In 1994, Dr. Wheeler was asked to serve as Chairman of Surgery at the Eastern Virginia Medical School. He then accepted an appointment in the same year as Dean and Provost where he served for five years. He retired in 1999 as Professor Emeritus of Surgery.

Dr. Wheeler died on April 13, 2024 at age 91. He was married for many years to Bonnie Martinette Wheeler who is a Masters prepared RN and also an attorney. Together they had five children, fourteen grandchildren and two great grandchildren.

Scan the QR code below or enter the YouTube link to watch the entire interview with Dr. Jock R. Wheeler conducted by Walter J. McCarthy, MD, and Roger T. Gregory, MD, brought to you by the SVS History Project Work Group.

 http://tinyurl.com/WheelerXJ

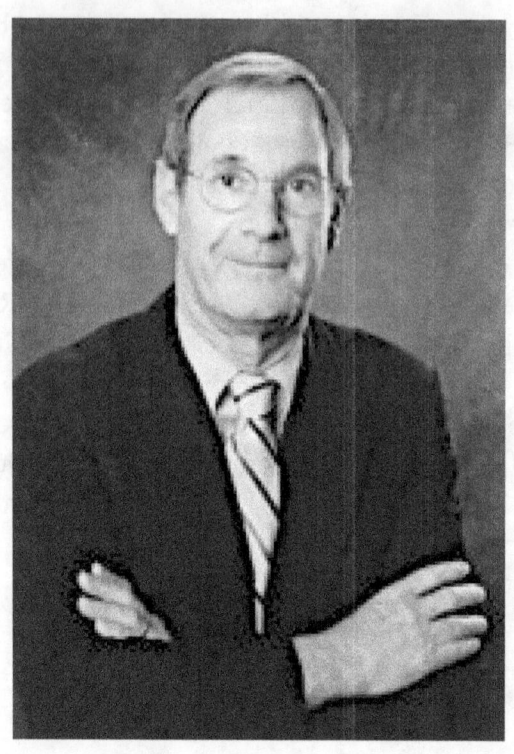

Anthony Dunster Whittemore, MD

Anthony Whittemore was born in Boston in 1944. Both sides of his family had lived in Massachusetts during the Revolutionary War. General Gansevoort, on his mother's side, served under George Washington, and among other interesting relatives on that side of the family, Dr. Whittemore also includes the author Herman Melville. Sam Whittemore, a farmer in Arlington, Massachusetts who was an ancestor on his father's side, had been too old to enlist in the Continental Army during the Revolutionary War. However, armed with only a pitchfork he was involved in a skirmish with British solders and nearly died of the retaliatory bayonet wounds.

Andy grew up in Cohasset, on Boston's south shore, and remembers being able to walk across the street to go sailing on Massachusetts Bay. During his youth, the experience of two family tragedies compelled Andy to consider studying medicine. His father, who had previously been a Navy pilot, died at age 38 when Andy was only 15 years old. Soon afterwards, his younger brother died of melanoma. The dual emotional shocks pointed Andy toward medicine as a career. It was something for which he had an natural aptitude as well. As a high school student, Andy enjoyed and excelled in biology and also met his future wife, who later become a nurse. They went to the senior prom together.

Over the years, Andy's entire family had attended Harvard—including one relative who was Harvard's first president, Henry Dunster—but Andy decided to strike out on a new path for his education. He was accepted prior to college to Columbia University's College of Physicians and Surgeons. He first earned a degree at Trinity College in Hartford, Connecticut without having to worry about getting into medical school. After medical school, Dr. Whittemore stayed at Columbia for five years of surgical residency, gaining good clinical experience at a number of New York City hospitals. His notable mentors included Arthur Voorhees, Ken Ford and Keith Reemtsma.

Having been deferred from military service until after completing his surgical residency by the Berry Plan, Dr. Whittemore then fulfilled his obligation with the U.S. Navy at the Portsmouth Naval Hospital in Norfolk, Virginia. Because of the great number of military retirees in that area, a multitude of vascular operations were needed. Dr. Whittemore's team had four residents on the service and he personally performed as many as 400 arterial reconstructions each year.

Since he and his wife were raised in the Boston area, following military service Dr. Whittemore jumped at the chance to work with Dr. John Mannick at the Peter Bent Brigham Hospital. There, he developed a vascular practice and focused his research on the role of synthetics for peripheral bypass and the biology of the arterial wall, as well as the evolution of vein graft stenosis. Thus, Dr. Whittemore began a decades-long association with Harvard Medical School, rising from Instructor in Surgery to Professor. He served as Chief of Vascular Surgery and Fellowship Director and also as Vice-Chairman of the Department of Surgery.

After many years and 15,000 surgical cases, Dr. Whittemore shifted his focus to administration, becoming Chief Medical Officer at the Brigham and Women's Hospital. He advocated for cultural change and modern measures such as barcoding medicines, which reduced errors by 50 percent.

Dr. Whittemore has participated in many domestic and international medical societies, serving as president of the International Society for Cardiovascular Surgery, the New England Society for Vascular Surgery, and the Boston Surgical Society. He was greatly honored to be named president of the American Surgical Association in 2008, following in the footsteps of his mentor, John Mannick, who had been president of that society in 1989.

Dr. Whittemore is a prolific writer who has authored hundreds of articles, reviews, chapters and editorials. He was also Editor-in-Chief of the ten-volume *Advances in Vascular Surgery*.

In an effort to maintain some normalcy in his life, he believed in always being home for dinner with his wife and three children, even if it meant working into the evening afterwards. Dr. Whittemore and his wife are proud grandparents of six grandchildren.

Scan the QR code below or enter the YouTube link to watch the entire interview with Dr. Anthony D. Whittemore conducted by Norman M. Rich, MD, brought to you by the SVS History Project Work Group.

 http://tinyurl.com/WhittXA

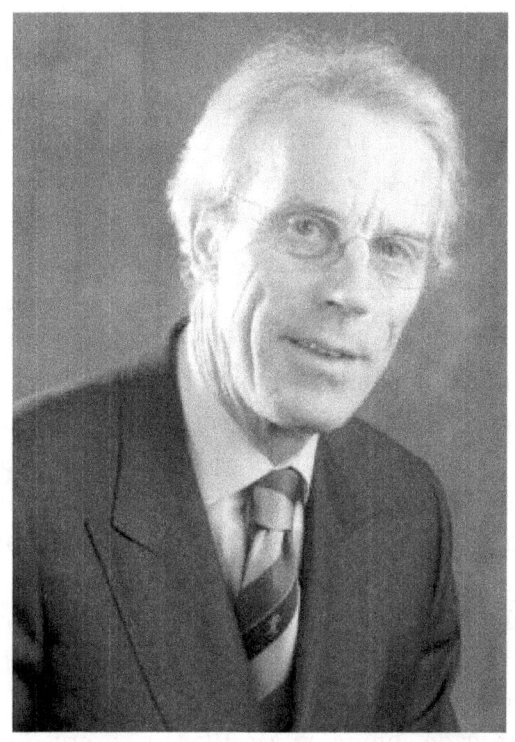

John H.N. Wolfe, MD

John H.N. Wolfe was born in Cardiff, Wales in 1947. His grandfather was a general practitioner, his mother a nurse and his father a surgeon. John's family moved to London in 1949, when his father received an appointment there. John attended boarding school in the south of England where he very much enjoyed rugby.

John was admitted to medical school at St. Thomas' Hospital in London, where he spent five years in what he remembers as intensely clinically-based training. He did his surgical internship at St. Thomas' as well, under Professor Frank Cockett (1916–2014). Professor Cockett is remembered for his contribution to vein surgery, including the three levels of perforating veins between the knee and the ankle, which now bear his name. After further studies at St. James' Hospital in Bristol, Mr. Wolfe worked as a registrar in Salisbury for 18 months. He then returned to St. Thomas' Hospital to work as a registrar and performed research with Professor John Kinmonth (1916–1982). Professor

Kinmonth was a pioneer vascular surgeon and a world authority on the lymphatic system. Therefore, Mr. Wolfe's thesis was written on lymphedema.

Mr. Wolfe then took a one-year research fellowship with Dr. John Mannick at the Peter Bent Brigham Hospital in Boston. Dr. Alec Clowes was at the Brigham at the same time as a clinical fellow, and the two fellows became life-long friends.

Throughout his career Mr. Wolfe has written more than 300 peer-reviewed articles and more than 100 book chapters. Early in his career, because of his thesis and knowledge of lymphedema, Mr. Wolfe was invited by Robert Rutherford to consult on the upcoming edition of Rutherford's textbook on vascular surgery. Mr. Wolfe's honors include being named a Hunterian Professor of the Royal College of Surgeons and a Moynihan Fellow of the Association of Surgeons of Great Britain and Ireland. Dr. Wolfe is known for his work advancing the visceral hybrid procedure for thoraco-abdominal aneurysms. This concept involves first bypass reconstruction of the visceral and renal arteries before endovascular stent graft repair of a thoraco-abdominal aneurysm. For teaching vascular technique he is very much a proponent of vascular training using vascular workshops and simulators.

Among his other leadership roles, Mr. Wolfe has served as president of the European Board of Surgery and as chairman of the European Training Committee of the European Society for Vascular Surgery. He was interviewed on June 18, 2015, at the Society for Vascular Surgery annual meeting in Chicago, Illinois. At that time Professor Wolfe was a Consultant Vascular Surgeon at St. Mary's Hospital in London.

Scan the QR code below or enter the YouTube link to watch the entire interview with Professor John H.N. Wolfe conducted by Roger T. Gregory, MD, and James S.T. Yao, MD, brought to you by the SVS History Project Work Group.

 http://tinyurl.com/WolfeXJ

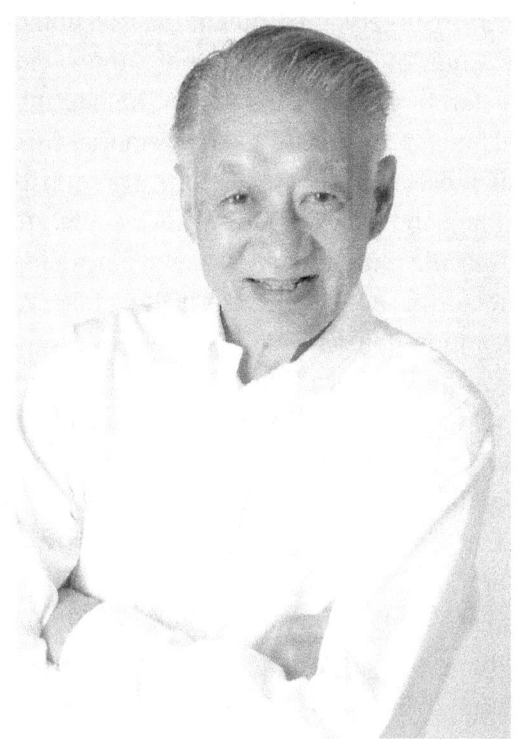

James S.T. Yao, MD, PhD

Dr. James S.T. Yao is world-renowned for his work with non-invasive vascular testing, which he advanced during his training at St. Mary's Hospital in London with Professor W.T. Irvine. The concept of measuring an ankle arterial blood pressure using Doppler ultrasound was the basis of his PhD thesis from the University of London and was published in the *British Journal of Surgery* in 1968. The resulting Ankle-Brachial Index (ABI) has become a simple, non-invasive test that provides physicians with a clear sense of a patient's condition without requiring complex imaging or scans.

After finishing his PhD, Dr. Yao was soon recruited to Northwestern University in Chicago by another young vascular surgeon, John J. Bergan. He founded the blood-flow laboratory at Northwestern Memorial Hospital in 1972. Dr. Yao remained at Northwestern for the rest of his career. By the time Dr. Yao had retired from clinical surgery as Emeritus Professor of Surgery at Northwestern's Feinberg School of Medicine, he had served Northwestern as the

Magerstadt Professor of Surgery, the Chief of the Division of Vascular Surgery (1988–1997) and the Chair of the Department of Surgery (1997–2000). Always respected as an outstanding technical surgeon, he had maintained a tremendously busy clinical practice at Northwestern Memorial Hospital for more than 35 years. One of his most important and enduring contributions to vascular surgery was the training and mentoring of young people, students, general surgery residents and vascular surgeon fellows. Not surprisingly, from 1972 until 1994 he was the director of the Northwestern University Vascular Fellowship, which he had helped to initiate.

James Yao was born in war-torn Canton, China, the region now known as Guangzhou, on October 14, 1934. Prompted by the Japanese invasion of China, his family moved to nearby Macao where Jim grew up.

He was a 1961 medical graduate of National Taiwan University Medical School. However, Dr. Yao found little opportunity for advanced training at home and thus sought general surgical training at Cook County Hospital in Chicago (1961–1967). Most notably, while at Cook County Hospital, Dr. Yao met Louise, who was a nurse at the hospital, and soon they were married. Together they have raised three children: Kathy, who is an oncology surgeon in the Chicago area, Pauline, an international art curator in Hong Kong, and John, a musician in New York City. After Jim graduated from general surgery at Cook County, the newlyweds traveled to St. Mary's Hospital Medical School in London.

Since his days of PhD training and throughout his Northwestern career, Dr. Yao's research interests have centered around surgical arterial and venous problems, non-invasive diagnostic techniques and basic, molecular issues related to aortic aneurysms. These investigations have formed the basis for more than 500 contributions to the surgical literature. In addition, he was co-editor of more than 50 books pertaining to vascular surgery, including two texts on non-invasive vascular diagnosis and one on angiography for vascular disease. He also served as co-editor of the annual *Year Book of Vascular Surgery* from 1986 to 1991.

Among his many leadership and academic roles, Dr. Yao served as president of the Lifeline Foundation, the Society for Vascular Surgery (SVS), the Midwestern Vascular Surgical Society, the Chicago Surgical Society and the American Venous Forum. He also served as an Associate Editor of the *Journal of Vascular Surgery* and the *Journal of Endovascular Surgery,* as an editorial board member of the *Annals of Vascular Surgery* and the *British Journal of Surgery,* and as co-chief editor (1996–2002) and later as chief editor of the journal *Cardiovascular Surgery* (2002–2003).

Dr. Yao has been honored with the Society of Vascular Technology Pioneer Award (1998), the Christian Fenger Award from the Karl Meyer Surgical Society/Surgical Alumni Association of Cook County Hospital (2003), the Society for Vascular Surgery's Lifetime Achievement Award (2007), and the Pioneers in Performance Award (2010). In 2015, Dr. Yao was awarded the René Leriche Prize by the International Society of Surgery. As a fitting tribute, September 21, 2005 was declared James Yao Day in Chicago by the city's mayor.

Jim Yao was always intrigued by history, both world history and in particular the history of vascular surgery. He was Co-Chairman of the SVS's 50th anniversary history presentation in 1997 with Calvin Ernst and was assisted by Bill Pearce. More recently, this led to his initiating and leading the SVS History Project Work Group, which is outlined by this book. The project, which began in 2011, has produced more than 90 video interviews of notable vascular surgeons. The organization, filming, editing and writing related to this huge project gave him tremendous satisfaction and enjoyment. He was still contributing to the work until several weeks before his death on December 20, 2022 at age 87.

Scan the QR code below or enter the YouTube link to watch the entire interview with Dr. James S.T. Yao conducted by Roger T. Gregory, MD, brought to you by the SVS History Project Work Group.

 http://tinyurl.com/YaoXJST

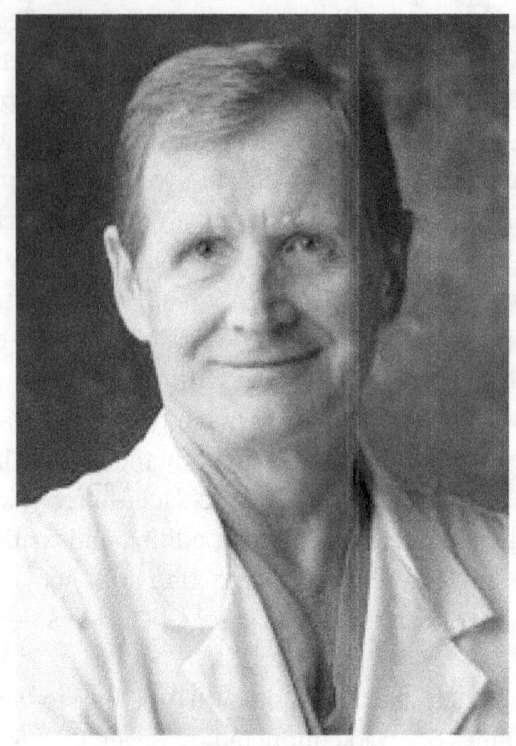

Christopher K. Zarins, MD

Christopher Zarins was born in Latvia on December 2, 1943, as World War II raged in Europe. At that time, his father was the minister of a major church in Riga, Latvia, which had been built in 1300. In October, 1944, Chris' family fled in a small boat across the Baltic Sea to Sweden, just ahead of the Soviet military occupation of their country. After World War II ended, the family moved from Sweden to the United States, and Chris' father was appointed to head a Latvian church in New York City. The year was 1946 and was just before a vast number of post-World War II Latvian refugees arrived at Ellis Island in New York harbor. Dr. Zarins' family helped many arrivals resettle in America.

Chris' mother was a teacher and strongly emphasized her children's education. Chris attended public schools PS77 and JHS51 in Brooklyn and graduated from Brooklyn Tech in 1960 during the excitement of the Sputnik era. Because he perceived a great need for engineers, Chris attended Lehigh University, initially planning to study engineering, but he finished with a bachelor's degree in biology. His interest in anatomy led him to medicine and Johns Hopkins University for medical school, where he was involved with many research projects, some involving animal surgery. Chris worked in the lab directed by David Skinner at Hopkins, who he identifies as his first great mentor, and graduated in 1968. Just before graduation, Chris met his wife-to-be, Zinta, at a Latvian community summer music and culture program.

Dr. Zarins completed his surgical residency at the University of Michigan where William Fry (1928–2007), his second great mentor, was practicing and teaching vascular surgery. At Michigan, Chris worked alongside several other future vascular surgeons—Jim Stanley, Pat Clagett and Jack Cronenwett—who were also residents at that time. From Dr. Fry, Dr. Zarins remembers learning the importance of high surgical standards and that patient care was the top priority.

Following residency, Dr. Zarins served in the US Navy for two years in San Diego, working in the Danag Shock Lung Unit. There, he did clinical research and critical care including learning about non-invasive vascular testing. After his military service, in 1976, Dr. Zarins was recruited to Chicago by Dr. Skinner, who by then was the Chief of Surgery at the University of Chicago. Dr. Zarins became the first full-time vascular surgeon on the faculty. He was named Chief of Vascular Surgery, built a clinical and vascular research program and founded the vascular surgery fellowship.

At the University of Chicago, Chris met his third great mentor, the pathologist Seymour Glagov. The two men made great inroads into changing the understanding of atherosclerosis by pooling information acquired in the OR, the animal lab and the morgue. The papers they produced together include many strikingly original observations. These include that arteries may compensate for stenosing atherosclerosis by increasing their external diameter. They also greatly increased our understanding of the relationship between arterial sheer stress and the location of atherosclerosis in arteries. It is not surprising that from 1983 until 1996, Dr. Zarins served as the editor of the *Journal of Surgical Research*.

After consulting with Stanford University, in 1993 Dr. Zarins accepted an offer to become Chief of Vascular Surgery at Stanford and to establish a vascular program and fellowship there. At Stanford, by combining the talents of Drs. Thomas Fogarty, Michael Dake and Charlie Taylor and the advanced imaging provided by Silicon Graphics computers, great strides were made in the understanding and treatment of occlusive arterial disease. In recent years Dr. Zarins has continued to refine this work through his company, HeartFlow, which uses computational flow analysis to aid in selecting the best course of treatment for patients.

Dr. Zarins' life came full circle when he returned to his birth country, Latvia, in 1986 for the first time since childhood for the World Congress on Biomechanics. At that time, Riga was the second leading center in the Soviet bloc, after Moscow, for the study of medicine. At the Congress Dr. Zarins made many connections with Latvian medical professionals, which led to a second major conference that he planned with his brother, an American orthopedic surgeon. This conference, called the World Congress of Latvian Physicians, took place in Riga in 1989 and was the first event where the new Latvian flag was raised. The pride instilled by the meeting, along with the collapse of the Soviet Union, contributed to the Latvian independence movement and resulted in a free Latvia in 1991. Dr. Zarins, his brother and his father were honored with the Three Star Order by Latvia in 2003 for their work on the Congress and also for their efforts in helping the new nation by organizing shipments of supplies and other donations.

This honor added to the achievements of a long productive career, balancing research and clinical practice, advancing knowledge of atherosclerosis and vascular modeling, which began in the labs at Johns Hopkins University and came to fruition at Stanford University.

In his presidential address to the Society for Vascular Surgery, which he delivered in June, 1999, Dr. Zarins provided this advice that truly has been reflected by his career: "Generate new knowledge, for knowledge will lead the way."

Scan the QR code below or enter the YouTube link to watch the entire interview with Dr. Christopher K. Zarins conducted by Melina R. Kibbe, MD, brought to you by the SVS History Project Work Group.

 http://tinyurl.com/ZarinsXC

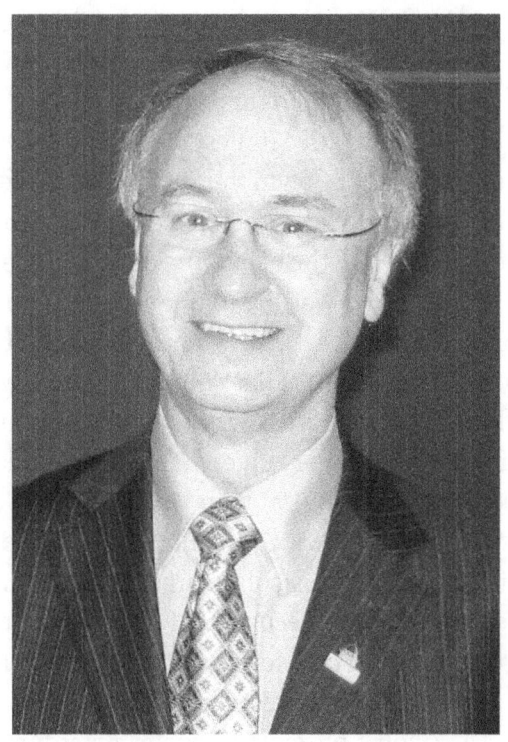

Robert M. Zwolak, MD

Robert Zwolak was born in 1948 in Bristol, Connecticut. His father was an entrepreneur involved in the automobile business, and his mother was a mortgage banker. Bob's early exposure to his father's businesses led him to an engineering degree at Rensselaer Polytechnic Institute in Troy, New York where he graduated in 1970.

Deciding to follow a more biological career, he took prerequisite courses for medical school, eventually earning a PhD. He subsequently graduated from Albany Medical School. There he was exposed to the well-known innovative trauma surgeon, Samuel Powers, whose example influenced Bob to select general surgery as a career path.

While interviewing for surgical residencies, Bob met with James Stanley at the University of Michigan and decided Michigan would be a perfect fit for him. While at the University of Michigan, Dr. Stanley's enthusiastic mentorship eventually led Dr. Zwolak to a vascular fellowship at the University of

Washington, where he trained under the tutelage of Eugene Strandness.

After fellowship, Dr. Zwolak was recruited to Dartmouth University by Jack Cronenwett and began practice there in 1987. Besides his busy vascular surgery clinical practice, administrative duties and teaching, Dr. Zwolak's career was also notable for his contribution to the Society for Vascular Surgery (SVS) and vascular surgery practice in general related to socioeconomic issues and government relations. He relates the beginning of these endeavors while working with Norman Hertzer (who was the SVS president from 1994 to 1995) during 1995 and 1996. At that time, representing the SVS, he began negotiating higher reimbursement rates for vascular surgery procedures with the Healthcare Finance Administration (HCFA). These activities continued and became a career-long contribution to vascular surgery. This included lobbying Congress, negotiating relative value units (RVUs) with HCFA (now called the Centers for Medicare and Medicaid Services, or CMS) and eventually developing a political action committee (PAC) for vascular surgery. The combination of these efforts has provided a tremendous economic boost to the profession of vascular surgery and to the quality of care for vascular patients through such things as the abdominal aortic aneurysm Medicare screening initiative.

For many years, Dr. Zwolak presented updates regarding national medical policy including coding and billing at the annual SVS meetings and became an extremely important expert resource for vascular surgeons. Dr. Zwolak eventually was honored as president of the Society for Vascular Surgery in 2011. As is often the case, he followed that position by being named President of the Vascular Surgery Foundation.

Scan the QR code below or enter the YouTube link to watch the entire interview with Dr. Robert M. Zwolak conducted by Roger T. Gregory, MD, and James S.T. Yao, MD, brought to you by the SVS History Project Work Group.

 http://tinyurl.com/ZwolakXR

Appendix I

It is important that the reader know something about the surgeons who conducted the interviews. Their background research and insights into the interviewee's circumstances and career details greatly enriched the conversations. All of the interviewers were members of the History Project Work Group and several of them, Drs. William Baker, Peter Lawrence, William Pearce, Norman Rich, and James Yao were themselves interviewed. The others who conducted interviews but were not interviewed are presented with biographies in the appendix for reference. These include Kenneth Cherry, Calvin Ernst, Mark Eskandari, Roger Gregory, Melina Kibbe, Richard Lynn, Walter McCarthy, and our videographer, Jan Muller. Two committee members, John (Jeb) Hallett and James Menzoian, were recruited at the very end of the project and never had an opportunity to conduct an interview.

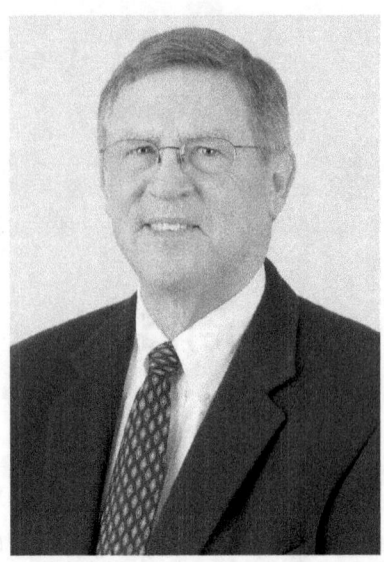

Kenneth J. Cherry Jr., MD

Dr. Cherry is currently Professor of Surgery at the University of Virginia (UVA) Health System in Charlottesville, Virginia. He was recruited there to become Division Chief of Vascular Surgery and Endovascular Surgery in January, 2004, and served in that role until 2010.

Dr. Cherry came to Virginia from the Mayo Clinic where he had practiced his entire career since 1981 and had served as the Chair of the Division of Vascular Surgery from April, 1990 until January 31, 2000. He was also Program Director for the vascular fellowship at Mayo for a number of years. During his more than 20 years at the Mayo Clinic, Dr. Cherry developed great expertise and became recognized as a world expert on a number of complex vascular surgery problems. These included surgical reconstruction for visceral ischemia and aneurysms and the management of thoraco-abdominal aneurysms. He also specialized in brachiocephalic and great vessel reconstruction, including cases related to Takayasu's arteritis. He was a noted authority on innominate artery reconstruction, carotid to subclavian artery bypass, and carotid endarterectomy surgery techniques. Based on the very extensive referral practice to the Mayo Clinic, Dr. Cherry and his partners at the Clinic—including Peter Pairolero, Larry Hollier, Jeb Hallett, Peter Gloviczki and Tom Bowers, among others—were able to publish many invaluable landmark papers related to vascular surgery treatment. This experience is reflected in Dr. Cherry's more than 190 published papers and 57 book chapters. It is noteworthy that in 2001 Dr. Cherry was asked to be the section editor for the Society for Vascular Surgery website on "expert techniques in open surgery."

When Dr. Cherry left the Mayo Clinic in 2004, he returned to Virginia, the state where he was born in Richmond on October 22, 1947. After high school, he had left Virginia for college at Duke, receiving a Bachelor of Arts in History in 1970. He then returned to the University of Virginia for his medical degree. Dr. Cherry stayed at the University of Virginia for a surgical internship and then general surgery training, finishing his chief residency in 1980. He had additional vascular surgery training at the University of California, San Francisco from July, 1980 until June, 1981 before being recruited to the Mayo Clinic as a young faculty member. In 1983, Dr. Cherry was in one of the first groups of young surgeons to receive recognition from the American Board of Surgery with a "Certification of Special Qualifications, General Vascular Surgery." This certification had first been offered in 1982.

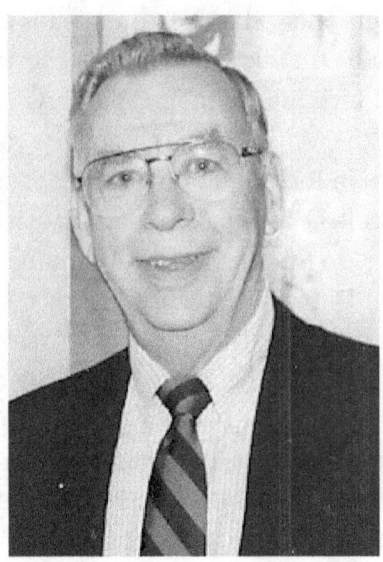

Calvin B. Ernst, MD

Calvin Ernst (1934–2015) was a prominent vascular surgeon in the United States who was present as a consultant at the very beginning of the History Project Work Group. He had previously worked on the 50th anniversary presentation for the Society for Vascular Surgery with James Yao. Dr. Ernst had served as the president of the Society for Vascular Surgery in 1990, and the History Project committee had intended to interview him because of that position. Unfortunately, he unexpectedly passed away on July 7, 2015 before he was interviewed. However, he can be seen face to face through this book and on video as he interviewed Harris Shumacker.

Dr. Ernst was born and raised in Detroit, Michigan, the son of a banker. He attended the University of Michigan for college, medical school (1959) and for his surgical residency. In addition, he joined the surgical faculty at the University of Michigan, but he left the faculty for a time during the Vietnam War, serving as a captain for two years in the U.S. Army from 1966 to 1968 with a MASH unit during the Tet Offensive.

After his military service, Dr. Ernst returned to the University of Michigan, but he was soon recruited to the faculty of the University of Kentucky and subsequently to the Johns Hopkins system in Baltimore. In 1985 he became the chief of vascular surgery at Henry Ford Hospital in Detroit, where he served for twelve years. Dr. Ernst finished his career at the Hahnemann School of Medicine in Philadelphia, from which he retired in 2000.

Besides his career-long clinical practice, where he was known as "a surgeon's surgeon," Dr. Ernst was a prolific contributor to the medical literature. He is well remembered for editing four editions of the outstanding text, *Current Therapy in Vascular Surgery*, with his friend, James Stanley. He co-authored 295 papers and book chapters during his career. Dr. Ernst was also a co-editor of *The Journal of Vascular Surgery* from 1991 to 1996.

Dr. Ernst's leadership skills led him to many important national positions, serving as the president of several surgical societies, including the Society for Vascular Surgery. He served a term as a director of the American Board of Surgery from 1991 to 1997.

Dr. Ernst met Elizabeth Thayer Abbott in college at the University of Michigan and they were married in 1957. They had four children.

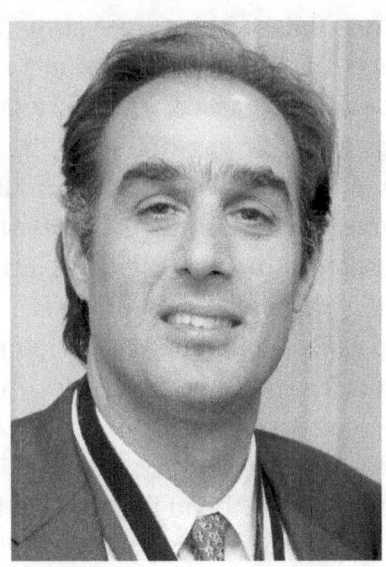

Mark K. Eskandari, MD

Dr. Eskandari has been a key part of vascular surgery at Northwestern University and the Northwestern University Medical Center in Chicago, Illinois for many years, since he was recruited in 1999 for his vascular fellowship. During his two-year fellowship he spent some of his time in the basic science laboratory where he was mentored by Dr. William H. Pearce, MD and Rex L. Chisholm, PhD. Dr. Eskandari was selected as the E. J. Wiley Traveling Fellow by the Society for Vascular Surgery in 2005. In 2010 he was honored to be named the first James S.T. Yao, MD, PhD Professor of Vascular Surgery, and that same year he was also appointed Chief of Vascular Surgery, a position in which he currently serves. In this position he is responsible for being Program Director of the vascular surgery training program and the course director for the Northwestern University vascular symposium. The symposium is held every December with an accompanying major textbook. Dr. Eskandari has served as the site principal investigator for a number of NIH-funded research initiatives including the Carotid Revascularization Endarterectomy vs. Stent Trial (CREST), 2002 through 2016. He also served as the co-investigator of the NIH Vascular Surgery Scientist Training Program, 2014 through 2019 at Northwestern. Additionally, he has been the investigator related to a large number of industry-funded research initiatives. Besides his extensive clinical practice, Dr. Eskandari has oversight responsibility for teaching, surgical care, funded research and faculty supervision over multiple campuses in the Chicago area. He has been honored with many teaching awards and is a member of nearly every important American surgical society, including the American Surgical Association, the Society of University Surgeons and the Society for Vascular Surgery.

Dr. Eskandari was born on January 21, 1966 and attended college (1984–1988) and medical school (1989–1993) at the University of Michigan. He went from Michigan to the University of Pittsburgh Medical Center for general surgery training, which he finished in 1999.

In the early 2000s, in his first years on the faculty at Northwestern, Dr. Eskandari was very influential in establishing a carotid artery stenting program and introducing techniques for endovascular management of the thoracic aorta. These, along with his many other vascular surgery interests, have resulted in more than 180 peer-reviewed papers and 70 book chapters. He also has been responsible for co-editing more than 18 textbooks, many of them related to the annual Northwestern vascular symposium.

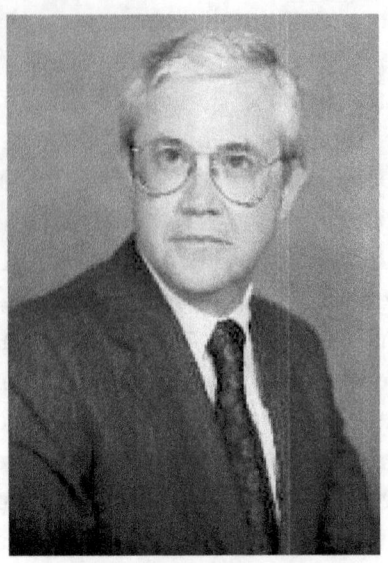

Roger T. Gregory, MD

Roger Gregory is Professor of Clinical Surgery at Eastern Virginia Medical School where he practiced vascular surgery, beginning as Instructor in Surgery there in 1973. He later became the chief of the vascular surgery division, and also director of the vascular fellowship program from 1994 until 2000. Dr. Gregory's career spans a period of rapid development in open vascular surgery, and, in fact, he is the surgeon who performed the first Gore-Tex femoral-popliteal bypass. Dr. Gregory was the primary surgeon, assisted by his partner and mentor Jock Wheeler, who performed this bypass with a 6 mm PTFE prosthesis on August 25, 1975.

Dr. Gregory's solid foundation and expertise with virtually every aspect of vascular surgery began with a fellowship in cardiovascular surgery during 1973 and 1974 at the Baylor College of Medicine in Houston, Texas. At the time Michael DeBakey was the chief of the service there. It is notable that 30 years later, Dr. Gregory was honored to be named President of the Michael E. DeBakey International Surgical Society in 2003–2004.

Born on July 17, 1939 in Rocky Mountain, North Carolina, Dr. Gregory traveled to Durham, to Duke University, for a Bachelor of Arts in Zoology, graduating in 1961. He then received his medical degree at the Medical College of Virginia in Richmond in 1965. He continued at the Medical College of Virginia for his internship and surgical residency, finishing in 1970. Because of the

Vietnam War, Dr. Gregory then entered the military and was assigned to the Arctic Medical Research Laboratory in Alaska. He authored several important papers on cold exposure based on that experience, including publications in *The Lancet* and *Surgery*. After discharge from the military, Dr. Gregory went on to his cardiovascular fellowship at Baylor and then was recruited to Eastern Virginia Medical School.

Besides his busy clinical practice and teaching responsibilities, Dr. Gregory is an inventor of surgical equipment having developed at least 14 different instruments or sets of instruments. These instruments are now produced by companies including Codman, Pilling, Lorenz and V. Mueller. Two of the best-known instruments are the "soft" carotid clamp (1975), usually referred to as a "Gregory Bulldog," and the perfectly shaped "Profunda" clamp (1980). The Profunda clamp is fourth from the left on the front cover of this book.

Dr. Gregory has been one of the main driving forces behind the current History Project Work Group which has expanded his career-long passion and natural skill for interview-based video recording of surgical history. His tenacity has been critical in keeping this long-term documentary project viable.

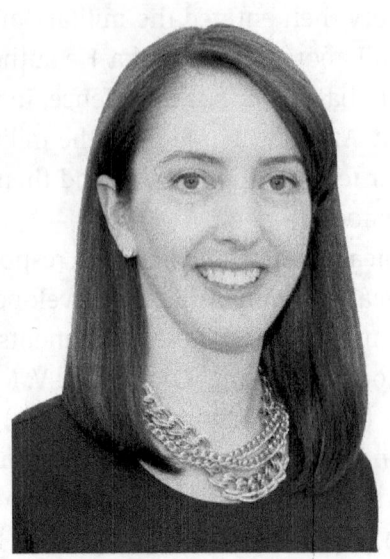

Melina R. Kibbe, MD

Dr. Melina Kibbe is the Dean of the University of Virginia School of Medicine. Dr. Kibbe's vascular fellowship (2002–2003) was at Northwestern University, after which she remained on the faculty until June 2016. During those years she also maintained a busy clinical service and directed a highly productive and funded basic science research laboratory.

Dr. Kibbe was born on May 15, 1968 in La Jolla, California, and was raised in Southern California. Her college (1990), and medical school (1994) education was at the University of Chicago. After medical school, Dr. Kibbe received all of her general surgery training at the University of Pittsburgh where she was exposed to the busy vascular surgery service there. Dr. Kibbe's research focuses on developing novel therapies to help patients who have vascular disease and to better understand the vascular wall itself. She currently is the author or co-author of more than 300 peer-reviewed papers and holds more than ten patents or provisional patents. Her research was recognized by President Obama with the "Presidential Early Career Award for Scientists and Engineers" in 2009. As a young faculty member at Northwestern, Dr. Kibbe became the chief of the vascular service at the Jesse Brown VA Medical Center and rose through the academic ranks to Professor of Surgery at Northwestern University. She obtained NIH and VA Merit Review and much other funding and also mentored numerous medical students and vascular trainees in her operating room and laboratory. At Northwestern Dr. Kibbe was named as the vice-chair of research in the department of surgery and Deputy Director of the Simpson Querrey Institute for BioNanotechnology.

Dr. Kibbe was recruited in 2016 to become the Chair of the Department of Surgery at the University of North Carolina, where she worked until 2021. During her career, Dr. Kibbe has received many national awards and teaching awards and has also been honored to be the president of the Association for Academic Surgery, the Midwestern Vascular Surgical Society and the Association of Veterans Affairs Surgeons. Notably, she was elected to the National Academy of Medicine in 2016. Dr. Kibbe has served as the Editor-in- Chief for *JAMA Surgery* for many years. Dr. Kibbe is also the co-founder and chief medical officer of VesselTek BioMedical, LLC, which works to develop medical devices for vascular disease.

On September 15, 2021 Dr. Kibbe became Dean and the James Carroll Flippin Professor of Medical Sciences at the University of Virginia Medical School where she is also Chief Health Affairs Officer at UVA Health.

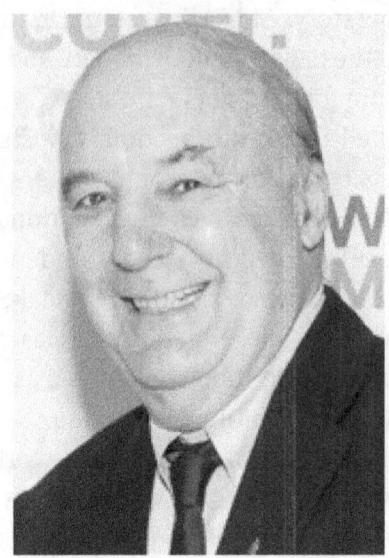

Richard A. Lynn, MD

Born in New York City, Richard Lynn attended New York University, where he graduated Phi Beta Kappa in 1967. Richard remained in New York City for medical school at Cornell University, finishing in 1971. He then completed his internship at the Harvard Medical School, Beth Israel Hospital in Boston. After medical school, he returned to New York City, to the Columbia University Roosevelt Hospital for general surgery training, completing his residency there in 1976. During the Vietnam War, Dr. Lynn also served as a captain in the US Air Force Reserve, based at the Westover Air Force Base in Massachusetts, from 1971 to 1973.

Beginning in 1976, Dr. Lynn began a private practice in vascular, endovascular, general and oncologic surgery in West Palm Beach, Florida, which he continued actively until 2013. He became affiliated with the Florida International University College of Medicine in Miami, first as a clinical assistant professor of surgery in 2008 and then as an associate professor of surgery in 2013.

Besides his busy clinical practice, Dr. Lynn has contributed significantly to a number of surgical societies. He has long been involved with the American College of Surgeons (ACS), where he was the president of the Florida Chapter in 2006–2008 and was honored as the second vice president of the main body of the ACS in 2021. Among his many committee contributions to the

ACS, particularly relevant to this book project, Dr. Lynn was a founding member of the ACS Surgical History Group.

Dr. Lynn has also contributed much to the Society for Vascular Surgery (SVS), helping the Political Action Committee, guiding the Community Practice Committee as Chairman for five years beginning in 2012, and serving on the SVS Board of Directors. He was a member of the SVS Foundation Board of Directors from 2017 until 2022. Dr. Lynn was recruited by Dr. Yao to be a member of the SVS History Project Work Group in 2015. Dr. Lynn served as the chief of surgery at several of the hospitals where he practiced in Florida and was also president of Temple Emanu-El in Palm Beach from 1984 until 1992.

Dr. Lynn has received many honors and awards related to his surgical practice and his contributions to organized medicine. These include the SVS Presidential Citation Award in 2016. He also received the SVS Excellence in Community Service Award, as the inaugural recipient in 2019. In 2017, an annual student scholarship at the Weill Cornell Medical College was established in Richard Lynn's name by grateful patients and community members in the Palm Beach area.

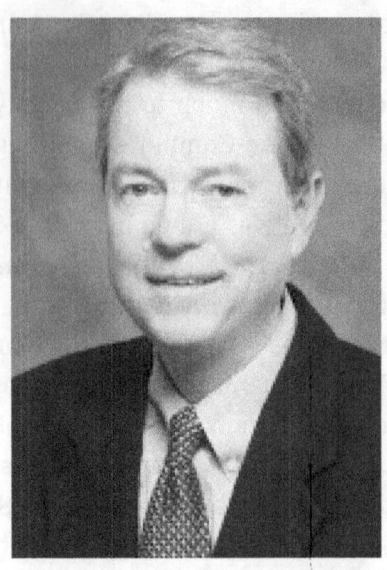

Walter J. McCarthy III, MD

Walter McCarthy received all of his surgical training, including a vascular fellowship (1983–1985) at Northwestern University. He then served on the faculty at Northwestern for 13 years, in practice with his mentors John Bergan, James Yao, William Flinn and William Pearce. In 1998, Dr. McCarthy was recruited to be Chief of Vascular Surgery at Rush University Medical Center in Chicago by Dr. Hassan Najafi. At Rush he also became the director of the vascular fellowship and for three years served as the chairman of vascular surgery at Cook County Hospital. He was Acting Chairman of the Department of Cardiovascular-Thoracic Surgery (2010–2013) during which time he was named as the John Bent Professor of Surgery. In those years he established a baccalaureate level program at Rush to train vascular ultrasound technologists. He also was instrumental in founding a physician assistant training program at Rush, and he served as Medical Director of both of these health-sciences programs over many years.

Dr. McCarthy has a career-long interest in lower extremity ischemia and tibial bypass surgery and also the management of intermittent claudication. He also is particularly interested in treating diseases of the thoracic aorta, including thoraco-abdominal aneurysm repair and in the descending thoracic aorta to femoral bypass operation.

Dr. McCarthy was born on August 14, 1952 in Oak Ridge, Tennessee, where his father, an engineer, was studying at the national laboratory. Dr. McCarthy was raised in Birmingham, Michigan, a suburb of Detroit, and graduated from Albion College (1974) in southern Michigan. After college, the rich surgical experience at Wayne State University Medical School in Detroit convinced him to select surgery as a career.

While at Northwestern, because of a growing interest in clinical outcomes research, Dr. McCarthy earned an MS degree in epidemiology from the Harvard School of Public Health. Around that time, he also served as secretary and then president (2006–2007) of the Midwestern Vascular Surgery Society. He has published more than 200 articles and book chapters along with three textbooks. Dr. McCarthy retired from clinical practice in 2022 and is currently Professor Emeritus at Rush, where an annual visiting professorship in his name was established that year.

Dr. McCarthy has always been interested in history, particularly of exploration, politics and military topics. He found that he shared this interest with Dr. Yao many years ago and thus was easily recruited to join the History Project Work Group in 2011.

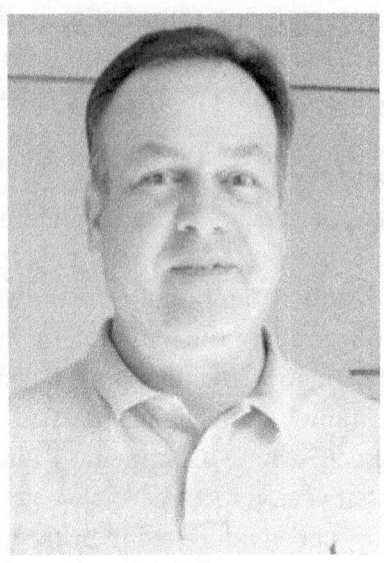

Jan Muller

Jan Muller is the videographer and video editor responsible for capturing and editing almost every interview produced by the Society for Vascular Surgery (SVS) History Project Work Group between 2011 and 2017. Mr. Muller was introduced to James Yao through a mutual friend and began the SVS project with nearly 25 years of previous video production experience. Just before the current project got underway, Mr. Muller had worked from 2001 until 2011 with Roger Ebert and Richard Roeper producing more than 500 episodes of their nationally syndicated movie review program, *Ebert and Roeper at the Movies* at WLS-TV in Chicago. This program, which had led Ebert to a Pulitzer Prize for criticism 25 years earlier, was a continuation of the already famous *Siskel and Ebert* program that had begun in 1975.

During Mr. Muller's part-time work with the SVS History Project he also spent much time as a freelance video editor for Exelon/Commonwealth Edison Creative Media, producing training and customer-outreach videos for the Chicago electric company. Mr. Muller was awarded two Midwest Emmys in 2013 and 2014 for editing *A Piece of the Game,* a nationally syndicated sports program.

During the recording of almost every History Project interview Mr. Muller worked with an assistant. This allowed for a two-camera style, one camera focusing on the interviewer and the other on the interviewee. Earlier interviews were recorded on DVCAM tape cassettes, and in later interviews digital single lens reflex cameras were used, which allowed transition to a wider screen image. Lavalier microphones were used for audio clarity. During editing, Mr. Muller integrated the soundtracks and video images to follow the conversations. Very notably, over the recording of more than 80 interviews in many different locations around the United States, none required re-filming due to any technical mishaps involving the audio or visual material.

Besides the video editing, Mr. Muller performed original research on topics mentioned during interviews and also incorporated photographs supplied by the interviewees related to their careers. He also not only edited written material but often authored biographical material himself or worked side-by-side on this with Dr. Yao.

The skills in all of these areas reflect Mr. Muller's early career background as a proofreader and writer following his graduation from Middlebury College as an English major in 1985. Before Middlebury, Mr. Muller was a 1981 graduate of Evanston Township High School in Illinois, where he was an honor student and standout in doubles tennis.

Appendix II

SVS HISTORY VIDEOS: DATES, LOCATIONS AND PARTICIPANTS
vascular.org/about/history

Enrico Ascher, MD
Interviewed by Kenneth J. Cherry, MD, & James S.T. Yao, MD; Vascular Annual Meeting (VAM), San Francisco, CA, 5/31/2013

Ronald J. Baird, MD
Interviewed by Walter J. McCarthy, MD; Northwestern Vascular Symposium, Chicago, IL, 12/9/2011

William H. Baker, MD
Interviewed by Walter J. McCarthy, MD; SVS Offices, Chicago, IL, 6/19/2012

Panagiotis E. Balas, MD
Interviewed by Norman M. Rich, MD, & James S.T. Yao, MD; VAM Boston, MA, 6/6/2014

Wiley F. Barker, MD
Interviewed by Peter F. Lawrence, MD; UCLA, CA, 2/20/2012

Jonathan D. Beard, MD
Interviewed by Roger T. Gregory, MD; Veith Vascular Symposium, New York, NY, 11/16/2012

Jean-Pierre Becquemin, MD
Interviewed by Walter J. McCarthy, MD, & James S.T. Yao, MD; VAM Chicago, IL, 6/18/2015

Ramon Berguer, MD
Interviewed by William H. Baker, MD; SVS Offices, Chicago, IL, 3/15/2012

F. William Blaisdell, MD
Interviewed by Norman M. Rich, MD; Stanford, CA, 1/11/2012

Jan D. Blankensteijn, MD
Interviewed by Walter J. McCarthy, MD, & James S.T. Yao, MD; VAM San Francisco, CA, 5/30/2013

Jan S. Brunkwall, MD
Interviewed by Norman M. Rich, MD; Veith Vascular Symposium, New York, NY, 11/15/2012

Jacob Buth, MD
Interviewed by Roger T. Gregory, MD, & James S.T. Yao, MD; VAM Boston, MA, 6/6/2014

Allan D. Callow, MD
Interviewed by Norman M. Rich, MD; San Francisco, CA, 10/17/2012

Richard P. Cambria, MD
Interviewed by William H. Pearce, MD, & William H. Baker, MD; SVS Offices, Chicago, IL, 10/1/2012

Piergiorgio Cao, MD
Interviewed by Walter J. McCarthy MD; VAM Boston, MA, 6/5/2014

Stephen W.K. Cheng, MD
Interviewed by Peter F. Lawrence, MD, & James S.T. Yao, MD; VAM San Francisco, CA, 5/30/2013

Timothy A.M. Chuter, MD
Interviewed by Roger T. Gregory, MD, & James S.T. Yao, MD; VAM Chicago, IL, 6/18/2015

G. Patrick Clagett, MD
Interviewed by Walter J. McCarthy, MD; VAM Washington, DC, 6/8/2012

Alexander W. Clowes, MD
Interviewed by Melina R. Kibbe, MD, & William H. Pearce, MD; SVS Offices, Chicago, IL, 9/11/2012

John E. Connolly, MD
Interviewed by Peter F. Lawrence, MD; UCLA, CA, 1/20/2012

Denton A. Cooley, MD
Interviewed by Roger T. Gregory, MD; Houston, TX, 9/26/2011

Jack L. Cronenwett, MD
Interviewed by William H. Baker, MD; SVS Offices, Chicago, IL, 6/1/2012

Herbert Dardik, MD
Interviewed by Melina R. Kibbe, MD; VAM Washington, DC, 6/8/2012

Richard H. Dean, MD
Interviewed by Mark K Eskandari, MD; Northwestern Vascular Symposium, Chicago, IL, 12/9/2011

DeBakey on Dr Matas
Michael E. DeBakey, MD; Interviewed by Roger T. Gregory, MD; Houston, TX

DeBakey on the SVS 50th Anniversary
Michael E. DeBakey, MD; Interviewed by F. William Blaisdell, MD; 1996

DeBakey Library/Museum Development Background
JoAnn Pospisil, MA, BA, & Mary Allen; Michael E. DeBakey Library/Museum, Houston, TX, 10/25/2016

DeBakey Library/Museum Project Background
James S.T. Yao, MD; Michael E. DeBakey Library/Museum, Houston, TX, 10/25/2016

DeBakey Remembered by Colleagues
Kenneth L. Mattox, MD, George P. Noon, MD, & Charles H. McCollum, MD; Interviewed by Roger T. Gregory, MD, Richard H. Lynn, MD, Walter J. McCarthy, MD, & James S.T. Yao, MD; Michael E. DeBakey Library/Museum, Houston, TX, 10/25/2016

DeBakey Library/Museum Tour
Conducted by Roger T. Gregory, MD, James S.T. Yao, MD, William T. Butler, MD, Kenneth L. Mattox, MD, George P. Noon, MD, & Charles H. McCollum, MD; Michael E. DeBakey Library/Museum, Houston, TX, 10/24/2016

James A. DeWeese, MD
Interviewed by James T. Adams, MD; Rochester, NY, 1999

Edward B. Diethrich, MD
Interviewed by Roger T. Gregory, MD, James S.T. Yao, MD, & Kenneth J. Cherry, MD; SVS Offices, Chicago, IL, 4/4/2013

Jeanne Doyle, RN
Victoria Fahey, RN
Interviewed by Walter J. McCarthy, MD, William H. Pearce, MD, & James S.T. Yao, MD; SVS Offices, Chicago, IL, 1/23/2017

Ben Eiseman, MD
Interviewed by Norman M. Rich, MD, William H. Pearce, MD, & W. Gerald Rainer, MD; Denver, CO, 5/31/2012

José Fernandes e Fernandes, MD
Interviewed by Kenneth J. Cherry, MD, & James S.T. Yao, MD; VAM San Francisco, CA, 5/31/2013

Thomas J. Fogarty, MD
Interviewed by Roger T. Gregory, MD, Melina R. Kibbe, MD, & James S.T. Yao, MD; SVS Offices, Chicago, IL, 5/25/2012

Julie Ann Freischlag, MD
Interviewed by Walter J. McCarthy, MD, Melina R. Kibbe, MD, with an introduction by James S.T. Yao, MD; SVS Offices, Chicago, IL, 2/6/2015

Peter Gloviczki, MD
Interviewed by Mark K. Eskandari, MD; SVS Offices, Chicago, IL, 3/14/2014

Olivier Goëau-Brissonnière, MD
Interviewed by Roger T. Gregory, MD, & James S.T. Yao, MD; VAM Boston, MA, 6/6/2014

Jerry Goldstone, MD
Interviewed by Kenneth J. Cherry, MD, & James S.T. Yao, MD; VAM San Francisco, CA, 5/30/2013

Richard M. Green, MD
Interviewed by Norman M. Rich, MD; VAM Washington, DC, 6/7/2012

Lazar J. Greenfield, MD
Interviewed by Peter F. Lawrence, MD; VAM Washington, DC, 6/7/2012

Roger M. Greenhalgh, MD
Interviewed by Roger T. Gregory, MD; Veith Vascular Symposium, New York, NY, 11/15/2012

John P. Harris, MD
Interviewed by Melina R. Kibbe, MD; VAM San Francisco, CA, 5/30/2013

Norman R. Hertzer, MD
Interviewed by Walter J. McCarthy, MD; SVS Offices, Chicago, IL, 9/5/2012

Larry H. Hollier, MD
Interviewed by Roger T. Gregory, MD; Veith Vascular Symposium, New York, NY, 11/16/2012

Jimmy F. Howell, MD
Interviewed by Roger T. Gregory, MD; Houston, TX, 8/23/2013

Anthony M. Imparato, MD
Interviewed by Roger T. Gregory, MD; NYU, New York, NY, 11/18/2011

Julius H. Jacobson II, MD
Interviewed by Roger T. Gregory, MD; NYU, New York, NY, 11/18/2011

K. Wayne Johnston, MD
Interviewed by Norman M. Rich, MD, & Peter F. Lawrence, MD; Veith Vascular Symposium, New York, NY, 11/16/2012

K. Craig Kent, MD
Interviewed by Peter F. Lawrence, MD; VAM Washington, DC, 6/6/2012

Robert L. Kistner, MD
Interviewed by Walter J. McCarthy, MD; SVS Offices, Chicago, IL, 6/25/2012

Peter F. Lawrence, MD
Interviewed by Walter J. McCarthy, MD, William H. Pearce, MD, & James S.T. Yao, MD; SVS Offices, Chicago, IL, 12/11/2015

Christos D. Liapis, MD
Interviewed by Norman M. Rich, MD, & James S.T. Yao, MD; VAM Boston, MA, 6/5/2014

Frank W. LoGerfo, MD
Interviewed by Melina R. Kibbe, MD, & James S.T. Yao, MD; SVS Offices, Chicago, IL, 5/12/2013

William T. Maloney
Interviewed by Norman M. Rich, MD, James S.T. Yao, MD, Jerry Goldstone, MD, Roger T. Gregory, MD, & Jonathan B. Towne, MD; VAM Boston, MA, 6/5/2014

John A. Mannick, MD
Interviewed by Roger T. Gregory, MD, James S.T. Yao, MD, & Walter J. McCarthy, MD; SVS Offices, Chicago, IL, 4/30/2013

Kenneth L. Mattox, MD
Interviewed by Roger T. Gregory, MD, & James S.T. Yao, MD; Houston, TX, 7/17/2012

James May, MD
Interviewed by Roger T. Gregory, MD, & Peter F. Lawrence, MD; Veith Vascular Symposium, New York, NY, 11/15/2012

D. Craig Miller, MD
Interviewed by Walter J. McCarthy, MD; SVS Offices, Chicago, IL, 3/26/2012

Frans L. Moll, MD
Interviewed by Kenneth J. Cherry, MD, & James S.T. Yao, MD; VAM San Francisco, CA, 5/31/2013

Wesley S. Moore, MD
Interviewed by Roger T. Gregory, MD; VAM Washington, DC, 6/7/2012

Hassan Najafi, MD
Interviewed by William H. Baker, MD, & James S.T. Yao, MD; Northfield, IL, 7/27/2012

George P. Noon, MD
Interviewed by Roger T. Gregory, MD; Houston, TX, 7/17/2012

John L. Ochsner, MD
Interviewed by Roger T. Gregory, MD; Jefferson, LA, 3/7/2013

Thomas F. O'Donnell, Jr., MD
Interviewed by William H. Baker, MD, & James S.T. Yao, MD; Northwestern Memorial Vascular Office, Chicago, IL, 7/26/2012

Juan Carlos Parodi, MD
Interviewed by Melina R. Kibbe, MD; SVS Offices, Chicago, IL, 5/1/2012

William H. Pearce, MD
Interviewed by Roger T. Gregory, MD; SVS Offices, Chicago, IL, 5/24/2012

Bruce A. Perler, MD
Interviewed by Walter J. McCarthy, MD, & Richard A. Lynn, MD; VAM San Diego, CA, 6/1/2017

Anatoly V. Pokrovsky, MD
Interviewed by Norman M. Rich, MD, & James S.T. Yao, MD; VAM San Francisco, CA, 5/31/2013

Jean-Baptiste Ricco, MD
Interviewed by Walter J. McCarthy, MD, & James S.T. Yao, MD; VAM San Francisco, CA, 5/30/2013

Norman M. Rich, MD
Interviewed by Roger T. Gregory, MD; Northwestern Vascular Symposium, Chicago, IL, 12/8/2011

Thomas S. Riles, MD
Interviewed by Roger T. Gregory, MD; VAM Washington, DC, 6/7/2012

Charles G. Rob, MD
Interviewed by Norman M. Rich, MD; Bethesda, MD, 5/21 & 6/18/1993

Harris B. Shumacker, MD
Interviewed by Calvin B. Ernst, MD; 1996

Gregorio A. Sicard, MD
Interviewed by Walter J. McCarthy, MD; SVS Offices, Chicago, IL, 4/19/2013

Anton N. Sidawy, MD
Interviewed by William H. Baker, MD, & William H. Pearce, MD; SVS Offices, Chicago, IL, 10/1/2012

Robert B. Smith III, MD
Interviewed by William H. Pearce, MD, & James S.T. Yao, MD; Atlanta, GA, 8/19/2013

Frank C. Spenser, MD
Interviewed by Roger T. Gregory, MD; NYU, New York, NY, 11/18/2011

James C. Stanley, MD
Interviewed by Walter J. McCarthy, MD, & James S.T. Yao, MD; VAM San Francisco, CA, 5/30/2013

Ronald J. Stoney
Interviewed by Norman M. Rich, MD; Stanford, CA, 4/2/2012

Jonathan B. Towne, MD
Interviewed by Walter J. McCarthy, MD; SVS Offices, Chicago, IL, 3/1/2012

Frank J. Veith, MD
Interviewed by Roger T. Gregory, MD; New York, NY

Frank J. Veith, MD
Interviewed by Roger T. Gregory, MD; Northwestern Memorial Vascular Office, Chicago, IL, 11/28/2012

J. Leonel Villavicencio, MD
Interviewed by Roger T. Gregory, MD; Northwestern Vascular Symposium, Chicago, IL, 12/9/2011

Shenming Wang, MD
Interviewed by Walter J. McCarthy, MD, Richard A. Lynn, MD, & Jinsong Wang, MD; VAM San Diego, CA, 6/1/2017

Milton Weinberg, MD
Interviewed by Walter J. McCarthy, MD, John V. White, MD, & James S.T. Yao, MD; Lake Forest, IL, 2/12/2016

Jock R. Wheeler, MD
Interviewed by Walter J. McCarthy, MD, & Roger T. Gregory, MD; Northwestern Memorial Vascular Office, Chicago, IL, 11/28/2012

Anthony D. Whittemore, MD
Interviewed by Norman M. Rich, MD; VAM Washington, DC, 6/7/2012

John H.N. Wolfe, MD
Interviewed by Roger T. Gregory, MD, & James S.T. Yao, MD; VAM Chicago, IL, 6/18/2015

James S.T. Yao, MD, PhD
Interviewed by Roger T. Gregory, MD; Northwestern Vascular Symposium, Chicago, IL, 12/8/2011

Christopher K. Zarins, MD
Interviewed by Melina R. Kibbe, MD; SVS Offices, Chicago, IL, 6/21/2012

Robert M. Zwolak, MD
Interviewed by Roger T. Gregory, MD, & James S.T. Yao, MD; VAM Boston, MA, 6/6/2014

www.ingramcontent.com/pod-product-compliance
Lightning Source LLC
Chambersburg PA
CBHW082035300426
44117CB00015B/2488